SOMEWHERE BETWEEN

Navigating the
Cancer Journey
with Faith

LINDY GORE

Somewhere Between: Navigating the Cancer Journey with Faith
by Lindy Gore

No part of this book may be used or reproduced in any manner, stored in a retrieval system, or transmitted in any form by any means—electronic, mechanical, photocopy, recording, or otherwise—without written permission of the author except as provided by United States of America copyright law.

Unless otherwise noted, scripture quotations are from THE HOLY BIBLE: NEW INTERNATIONAL VERSION ®, NIV® Copyright © 1973, 1978, 1984, 2011 by Biblica, Inc. ® Used by permission. All rights reserved worldwide.

The ESV® Bible (The Holy Bible, English Standard Version®). ESV® Text Edition: 2016. Copyright © 2001 by Crossway, a publishing ministry of Good News Publishers. The ESV® text has been reproduced in cooperation with and by permission of Good News Publishers. Unauthorized

Reproduction of this publication is prohibited. All rights reserved.

Scripture quotations noted NKJV are from the New King James Version®. Copyright © 1982 by Thomas Nelson. Used by permission. All rights reserved.

Holy Bible, New Living Translation, copyright © 1996, 2004, 2015 by Tyndale House Foundation. Used by permission of Tyndale House Publishers, Inc., Carol Stream, Illinois 60188. All rights reserved.

Copyright © 2022 by Lindy Gore
All rights reserved.

ISBN 979-8-9866586-1-2

Cover and Interior Design and Formatting: Rina Waligo (www.rinawaligo.com)
Cover and Interior Image Design: Reina Jenkins
Editing: Daltyn Terpstra

This book is dedicated with love to my husband,

Dave, the joy of my heart and my hero.

What Others Are Saying

This Holy Spirit inspired devotional is a must read for all women, not only those dealing with breast cancer. Lindy's vulnerability and transparency in the details of the physical and emotional challenges she faced bring a heightened awareness to families and friends of those battling cancer. Lindy not only shares her story, but also uses her teaching gift to link her experiences to Biblical examples. She weaves her quirky humor and deep love for the Lord into many of her writings and brings even the most fearful and dreadful experiences back to the goodness of God and hope for complete healing. Her positive voice and authentic faith shine light into the darkness of a difficult season. Reading this devotional is time well spent!

Sindy Nagel
Inspirational Author and Speaker

Faith in God and the perspective you carry are two of the most important aspects of facing a difficult trial. After personally observing Lindy navigate her cancer journey with an astonishing measure of joy, peace and faith, I knew she had a life changing message to share with the world! *Somewhere Between* is a compelling combination of relatable stories, devotions and prayers that will drive your faith, encourage you and let you know you're not alone. Lindy's raw honesty and vulnerability provides language to help you process your own journey and propel you to fight the good fight with confident faith.

Monica Lee
Groups Pastor, Radiant Church

In this inspirational devotional, Lindy leads us through her cancer journey while never losing sight or trust in her faith or in the infinite grace, mercy and compassion of Jesus Christ. She even adds some humor along the way to lighten the load -- which we all need. She offers a way to grow through this hard time. I would personally recommend *Somewhere Between* to anyone on the cancer journey.

Margaret McGovern
Founder, Cancer Hope Connections

This unique devotional highlights Lindy's personal account with God during her diagnosis and treatment of cancer. Skillfully threaded through this work is the emotional and spiritual struggle she's faced. Like David who cried out to God when he was overwhelmed, Lindy is brutally honest in confronting her Father with her fears, frustrations and delayed answers to prayer. She is just as honest about her own human failings and murmurings-something we can all relate to. In the end, it's her faith and trust in Him that trumps every twist in the road. Lindy's natural spontaneous language reads like talking to a friend. It's a wonderful book that will touch many lives.

Fleur Vas
Author and Editor

Contents

Acknowledgments	1
Foreword	4
Introduction	7
Day 1: Somewhere Between	14
Day 2: Embracing The Truth	19
Day 3: Patience in Waiting	24
Day 4: Listening for the Holy Spirit's Voice	30
Day 5: Sheltered in His Presence	35
Day 6: Old Command, New Ink	41
Day 7: Never Alone	46
Day 8: Singing in the Storm	50
Day 9: A New Thing	55
Day 10: Suspect Faith	59
Day 11: Levity Before Surgery	65
Day 12: Deconstruction	69
Day 13: Loss and Wholeness	74
Day 14: The Pitfall of Pride	79
Day 15: For Better or Worse	85
Day 16: Fight My Battles	91
Day 17: Beautiful in its Own Time	96
Day 18: No Worries	101
Day 19: Expanding	106
Day 20: Are You Willing?	111
Day 21: Awareness	116
Day 22: Unending Praise	122
Day 23: Privacy	126
Day 24: Marked by the Spirit	132
Day 25: No Shame	137

Day 26: Just Breathe	143
Day 27: Give Thanks	148
Day 28: Waiting for the Promise	152
Day 29: Ring the Bell	156
Day 30: Seize the Day	161
Day 31: Walkie Talkie	166
Day 32: Scars	171
Day 33: Intimacy	177
Day 34: Connection	182
Day 35: Leftovers	187
Day 36: Copays	192
Day 37: The Exchange	197
Day 38: Unexpected	201
Day 39: Hospital Hoopla	206
Day 40: Room for Others	211
Day 41: Stay in Step	216
Day 42: Gratitude	221
Day 43: COVID and Caregiving	226
Day 44: Build Up	231
Day 45: New Year Old Truths	235
Day 46: Hope in the Crushing	240
Day 47: Using Wisdom	245
Day 48: Checking In	249
Day 49: Prosthetics	254
Day 50: Sabbath Rest	259
Conclusion	265
Photo Collage	269
Appendix:	273
About The Author	279
Notes	281

Acknowledgments

When a book gets published, everyone is excited for the author. Truth be told, I've had a lot of inspiration, encouragement, mentoring, and professional help along the way. I always hesitate to name names for fear of leaving someone out, so if you are one of the unnamed, please forgive me and know that I appreciate everyone who has poured into me during this journey.

My greatest desire is to give all the glory to God for giving me a new life in Christ and putting His Spirit in me, enabling me to participate in what He's doing in the world. Without a relationship with Jesus, my words would be meaningless. It is only because of Him that this book was written at all.

I want to thank my amazing husband, David Gore, for not only being there every step of the way, but for giving me the dignity of making my own treatment decisions. He always pointed me to Jesus and showed me daily what it looked like to have the heart of the Father. I also want to acknowledge our extended families, who never stopped praying for us and believing for my healing. A special thanks to Ted and Dawn for their amazing hospitality during my radiation treatment and to my mom, who spent hours pre-editing before it ever went to a professional editor. I am forever grateful to my daughter, Lacey, for all the love, time, and the sacrifices she made for me during my illness, not to mention the countless prayers she sent to Heaven on my behalf.

There are so many dear Christian sisters to acknowledge, some of whom are also cancer survivors. They have poured into my life, brought food, cleaned my house, sent cards, and shared both tears and laughter with me along the way. A heartfelt thank you to Becky, Paula, Kim, Sindy, Sally, Margaret, Sandi, Cindy E, and Monica. What an amazing bunch of women you are! I love you all to pieces!

My sincere appreciation goes to the entire staff of Rogel Cancer Center at the University of Michigan. A special thanks to my "Cancer Killers" in Radiology Oncology and to Dr.

Jessica Hsu and her staff in the Plastics Department. You're the best teams on the planet!

Finally, I'd like to thank my amazing editor, Daltyn Terpstra, for making my words convey my heart, my cover designer, Reina Jenkins, for her brilliantly creative work, and Rina Waligo, for her tireless dedication, doing all the technical garbage I'm so terrible at. You've all helped this dream become a reality! To God be the Glory!

Foreword

It was the day before Thanksgiving. My to-do list was long: work, groceries, cooking, and a pesky mammogram, squeezed in (no pun intended) on this short workday. I adore tradition. Every year, I look forward to this day, minus the mammogram part. I love the smell of apples and cinnamon, the colors of the season, magnificent and fiery. I get giddy pulling my special holiday, big bowls from the recesses of their basement hiding place. There are a million precious details about all this that flood me with joy. But, in all my mind's wonderings, in all my thoughts for the day, in all my forward thinking, I could not have dreamed that in one moment, I would be plucked from my warm, fragrant, pumpkin-filled existence and harshly hurled into a new world: cold, sterile, technical and terrifying. I did not know with a few words from a technician, my life would shift. Good and bad, I would be forever changed.

Everyone has a journey. I never imagined cancer would be part of mine. Cancer is consuming - much more than just physically invasive. It leaves no part of you untouched. It changes you. Changes what you treasure - how you relate to yourself and others. Morphs what you see in the mirror. It can leave you gutted on the floor, or chisel you into a hardcore, championship fighter. Cancer causes you to value things you never noticed and question things you built your life upon. Cancer is a master teacher. I have learned things I didn't want to know and gleaned lessons that have made me a richer, more compassionate soul.

This book is a gift. My friend, Lindy, is the strongest, bravest woman I know. Over the years she has walked me through many dark seasons, including cancer. She is straightforward, insightful and refreshingly real. She is unafraid to address things from which others turn away. Her heart beats for people and you will feel it in her words. Her journey has inspired me and made me ugly cry. I have seen what cancer has done to her, and how her tenacious faith leads in her fight. You will get to know her in these pages, and it will be easy to understand why I am so grateful she is my friend. Whether this is your journey or the journey of someone you love, you will find true and useful insight in these pages. On the days you need it most, you will realize there is someone who understands.

Kimberly Rude,
Worshiper and Pink Sister

Introduction

It might sound dramatic, but I've seen what feels like all ends of the earth. Skydiving in Hawaii with the Pacific Ocean beneath my feet, camping on the plains of the Serengeti desert alongside baboons and wildebeests, walking the beaches at sunset in Thailand, zip lining from the top of the Great Wall in China, and floating in the salty water of the Dead Sea. This adventurous life is one that I am blessed to have experienced — more than most people will in their entire life. In all of this time traveling, there is one place I never dreamed of visiting, one I have not-so-affectionately named "cancer land." And to make it worse, this wasn't a short-term destination for me — I found myself experiencing an extended stay with no checkout in sight. Of all those experiences in life across many cities, countries, and continents, my cancer journey — the one that happened at home — taught me the most about myself, my priorities, my marriage, my faith, and the art of perseverance. Cancer is a "God journey" in the truest sense of the word. For those who find themselves experiencing "cancer land" or traveling as a companion to someone on this journey, prepare yourself. Your experience, as mine did, will teach you more about yourself and God than you know.

In July 2020, I was diagnosed with invasive breast cancer. (As if the worldwide pandemic wasn't enough for that year!) A year prior, I had gone in for a routine exam with my primary care physician. During the breast exam portion, she asked a question that evoked equal feelings of nervous laughter and doubt. She paused, asking "Have you always had an inverted nipple?" Through little giggles, I admitted I wasn't too sure. I wasn't subscribed to the regular at-home breast exams or paid too much attention to my body in that way. I mean, I basically missed my menopause experience because I was too busy with other things to take notice. Continuing the exam, she said she didn't feel anything abnormal but recommended a mammogram as soon as possible.

Following her directions, my 2D mammogram came back normal. *Phew! Some people have innies, some have outies, some must also have inverted nipples. Crisis averted.*

Introduction

Fast forward to June, 2020. With more time on my hands due to the world being shut down, I was taking a closer look and noticed that maybe what I had going on wasn't so normal after all. My nipple looked even more inverted and now my breast seemed misshapen. *Is this part of growing old? I am nearly sixty!* At the same time, I noticed an ache deep in my chest, but it was only mild so I tried to ignore it. In the middle of the pandemic, I still felt the need to try and schedule my yearly exam and mammogram — so I made the call and went to my appointment.

As with the year prior, there was still no lump of any sort, but with the changes to my nipple and breast shape, she recommended a diagnostic mammogram with 3D imaging. *No lump, no cancer, right? Just a routine check. It'll come back just fine!* I felt so confident, in fact, that when my husband, Dave, offered to go with me to the appointment, I said no. I had no angst about it at all, no thought that I could have cancer or was inches away from stepping into this arena.

Somewhere Between

What was supposed to be your typical boob-crushing, in-and-out mammogram turned into back-to-back appointments with the addition of an ultrasound to get even more imaging. *This is a lot of work for someone who doesn't even have cancer.* In between appointments, it still hadn't really clicked that maybe, just maybe, I did have something to worry about. I called Dave to let him know I'd be longer than I expected. Once again, he offered to come and meet me, and I said no. The second appointment, an ultrasound, was painless and easy. They took a series of pictures of my left breast from different angles. You would've thought they were making a scrapbook. I sat and waited in the room, fully expecting them to say all was well and I could go home. "See you next year!" was all I hoped to hear.

Five minutes, then ten minutes passed. For the first time in the day, I started to worry. I could feel the lump in my throat forming. After what felt like an eternity, the technician returned — with a friend. He introduced himself as the radiologist on staff and I can vividly remember my response. "Is this going to be bad news? Because if it is, I need to call my husband and have him listen in on speaker phone." He nodded somberly and my

Introduction

fingers hit my speed dial. He then went on to explain he had been doing this for many years and that even without a biopsy, he was 90% sure this was cancer. At that moment there was no fear. I could feel nothing; I was numb. I didn't understand. There was no lump. *No lump, no cancer, right?*

The cancer that had grown in my body wasn't forming a lump. It had spread in an area located just beneath my nipple, making it hard to see and nearly impossible to feel. The way to confirm was to take a biopsy, which we did. The results came back in just a few days to confirm what I had never believed to be possible: I had cancer.

For years, I've felt a little tug from the Lord to write. I've written some, maybe short stories or things for my kids, but had never taken the time to be truly obedient and seriously write. After my fourth surgery, I was told I needed to be completely still for a solid six weeks if I wanted to avoid skin grafts and other painful procedures. So, I sat, and when I sat, I found the time to write! I started by reading through my personal journal and CaringBridge updates. It didn't take long to figure out what

God wanted me to write about. It was heavy on my heart and very evident that He wanted me to write a devotional full of encouragement for other people going through their own cancer journey. True to that calling, this devotional is meant to encourage you with stories from my journey while sharing Biblical insights and lessons learned along the way. Your journey is unique to you, as is mine. Regardless of our individual diagnosis, we share similar experiences, emotions, and questions. As a believer, I look to my faith to find answers and comfort in the darkest of times — and celebrate times of victory by giving God the praise He deserves.

So, this devotional is made for you! I recommend you read it one day at a time. Even though it may not be exactly like your story, I hope that you will find pieces that resonate with you. Pray and ask the Holy Spirit what He wants to tell you through the reading, devotional, or prayer. Find ways to make it your own. Get a journal and write your own story, draw pictures, or sing your own anthems as you go through this journey. God wants to do something in and through you during this time. He

Introduction

won't waste a single minute of it, even when it feels like the whole thing is a waste.

Even before cancer, we were survivors. We survived things like childhood trauma, living with an addict, divorce, or single parenting. We survived years of supporting our families with both good and bad jobs, as stay-at-home moms, or in service to others. Personally, I've been through all these challenges and have also fought this new battle with cancer. Small but mighty, I hope this devotional will help you to survive and thrive regardless of where you are in your cancer journey. Just remember this: God is with you. He loves you and will give His best blessing to you and your family wherever it takes you.

Blessings and Hope

∽ DAY 1 ∾

Somewhere Between

Since 2020, some would say the most dreadful "c" word is COVID, but for me – it was cancer. Nearly everyone knows someone who is battling it, has survived it, or lost their life to it. Cancer is a sneaky guest taking up an unwelcome residence, rearranging the normal order of things and leaving absolute chaos in its path. No one really wants to deal with the havoc that cancer creates, and worst of all – ignoring its existence won't make it go away. Eventually, it must be confronted.

🎗 My Journey

No one expects to experience cancer and I am no different. Quite honestly, it still hasn't sunk in. When I saw reports that said an "invasive mammary adenocarcinoma" was growing in my left breast, they were simply just words on paper. They didn't seem true. *It can't be. Not me. Not now.* I felt fine except

Day 1: Somewhere Between

for a mild ache in my chest. My breast looked a little misshapen, but what middle-aged woman didn't think things looked a little wonky sometimes? I was tested, then tested again – mammogram, ultrasound, biopsy, CT scan, genetic testing. *This all seems like a stupid mistake.* I had been referred for a consultation with an experienced surgeon and yet still wasn't fully convinced of my new reality.

I walked into the Bronson Cancer Center for the first time and the thoughts started racing. *What am I doing here? I don't belong here with all these sick people. They're probably all wondering why I'm here, too. Why am I here?* The longer I sat there waiting for my name to be called by the kind nurse in blue scrubs, the more the uncomfortable feelings sank in. *When I leave here and get in my car to go home, I'll get my "real" life back. I'm a strong, healthy Iowa girl. These test results aren't right. They can't be!* Now I know, I was not alone in those feelings. It takes time for facts and feelings to align, and cancer doesn't work on our timetable. I wasn't at all interested in waiting to see this alignment come to fruition. I didn't want any of this to be real.

✷ Devotional

The first phase of dealing with any kind of trauma or loss is denial. No one wants to recognize the painful realities in their life. It is so much easier to believe that someone made a mistake, and the event or diagnosis is just a long, bad dream. As soon as we wake up, we think the nightmare will be gone. We want to believe once we shake off the cobwebs, everything will go back to normal – but unfortunately, that is rarely the case.

The Bible tells us that original sin corrupted God's perfectly created world and resulted in a broken relationship with God. In Genesis 3, Adam and Eve disobeyed God, blaming each other, and even God Himself, for their disobedience. Unfortunately, this made sin, sickness and brokenness our never-ending reality. Sin has a unique way of affecting every part of our lives and even if we haven't had a direct part in causing it, the fallout can impact us.

Day 1: Somewhere Between

Denial is our way of pushing the diagnosis away and refusing to truly acknowledge the ugliness of cancer. For some of us, denial can last a long, long time. We disassociate with both facts and feelings, simply because they're too painful to bear. It takes time to wrap our minds around the truth, but eventually we are forced to acknowledge it. While cancer may be our current reality, there is a greater reality at play. Through Christ, the bonds of sin and sickness are broken and as we walk with Him in this journey, we will be overcomers!

Prayer

Father, in the beginning, I know the world was not as it is today. You created all things to be perfect, beautiful, functional, and glorifying to You. I don't want to see or believe that this sickness is my reality. Thank You, Lord, for a gentle revelation of the truth, even when it's hard to swallow. Thank you for Your whispers of comfort and hope as I slowly awaken to the situation in front of me. Be merciful with me as I come into these new realities and hold me closely in Your loving embrace. I pray this in Jesus' name. Amen.

∽ DAY 2 ∽

Embracing The Truth

This afternoon, I found myself standing in front of my refrigerator, ravenously searching for something to eat. My hungry eyes lasered in on a container full of big, beautiful green grapes. I grabbed the entire container, tossing a handful in my mouth without even so much as a thought. What was expected to be an explosion of sweet, fruity flavor was quickly met with a jolt of sour squishiness that sent me running to the garbage can a few steps away. *Yuck! When did I buy these?*

In reflecting on that experience, I realized that there is something similar about those green grapes and my new reality as a cancer patient – seemingly fine on the outside with an unsuspected decay brewing on the inside.

Somewhere Between

🎗 My Journey

In my situation, I've felt physically strong with normal aches and pains caused by an aging body. I have no reason to believe anything is wrong – except a diagnosis from my doctor. When I looked at the test results, I remember thinking *"What the what?"* I saw pages full of long, jumbled medical jargon – many of them words I can't even pronounce! It sent me into a downward spiral of Google searches and nights pouring over medical journals seeking answers, explanations, and treatment plans. The goal? To gain understanding and ultimately, feel in control. The key word here: *feel.* I'm not truly in control of this at all, but I sure want to be.

Knowledge is power, right? Black and white medical information can help us understand the issues we face and make educated decisions alongside our healthcare providers. A search engine – yes, even Google – has no idea what other circumstances or individual components are working together to help or harm your particular situation. No situation is the

Day 2: Embracing The Truth

same and words in and of themselves cannot provide a full picture. The job of doctors is to analyze the information and give their best recommendations, but they are not able to account for what cannot be seen, understood, or measured by technology. Human wisdom has a report, but so does the Lord!

Devotional

In Numbers 13 & 14, we read the story of Moses sending out twelve leaders to scope out the land of Canaan. Ten of the twelve spies came back to report that the opposition was too great and very strong. They reported feeling like "grasshoppers in their own sight" and in the sight of the enemy. Joshua and Caleb, the other two spies, stood up to say they could take on the opposition to claim this land as their God-given inheritance.

Just like the ten spies, doctors and professionals are tasked to give a report based on what they see. But then, what does faith say? As believers, we understand that there are things that only God knows, can see, and can do. We can look at the medical reports, and easily feel defeated, but faith in our good Father will never be overshadowed by human wisdom. Thankfully, stating the facts does not determine the future. Our future is solely up to the Lord. Every day of our lives was written before even one of them ever came to be, so He and He alone determines our future. We pray daily for complete and total healing and are absolutely convinced it can happen.

Remember: we have an all-powerful God! We are also aware of our human state, somewhere between the "already accomplished" work of Jesus on the cross and the "not yet" full manifestation of His glory. As we sit in the physical and spiritual in between and wait for Him, we must continue to speak God's blessing over our lives. We stand fast in this truth. By His stripes we are healed!

Prayer

Father, You are sovereign. You are good. You have a good plan for my life and know it fully from beginning to end and everything in between. When words and facts overwhelm me

Day 2: Embracing The Truth

and paint a picture of reality that speaks negativity and death into my life, I come against it in Jesus' name! I declare that You and You alone are the author and finisher of my faith, and my life is directed by You. Help me, Lord, to live by faith. I know You can do exceedingly, abundantly more than I can ask or imagine. Speak life into me today as I seek to follow You more closely. In Jesus' name, Amen.

∾ DAY 3 ∾

Patience in Waiting

(With or Without Marshmallows)

In the 1960s, there was a study done called "The Marshmallow Test."

A group of four-year-olds were tested individually, left unsupervised in a room with a single marshmallow placed in front of them. The rules were simple. They could either eat the one marshmallow now or wait a little longer and get two marshmallows. Can you guess what the results were? They were hilarious and very telling of our innate ability to wait. The study continued for decades later, and eventually discovered that the children who were willing to wait for a greater reward were more likely to find traditional success in life (think: a four-year college degree or earn a high income). Even at that young age, we could measure the amount of self-control that a person

Day 3: Patience in Waiting

has – with something as simple as a marshmallow. As we age, the hope is that we gain more patience but the irony in developing patience is that it takes so incredibly long!

❦ My Journey

Remember all those tests I had to take? Well, I think waiting on the results would have been a lot easier if I had some marshmallows to snack on. It felt like an eternity. When the results started trickling in, the next task – trying to make sense of them – was even more daunting. Here I was, left with a thousand questions about medical terms, desperately wishing I knew enough to understand what is happening in my body on a molecular level. One of the tests that I was most anxious to get the results of dealt with gene mutation, and thank God it came back with nothing. This meant that my cancer wasn't something passed to me genetically and it also wasn't something that I could pass onto my children or grandchildren. One less burden, one less thing to feel guilty about, and I was grateful for a moment of relief. *Thank You, Jesus!*

Next, I received results from my more sensitive MRI scan. Unfortunately, this test had detected additional satellite cancer cells which had unexpectedly spread deeper into my breast tissue. *Where else could this cancer have gone?* So far, my doctors hadn't discovered cancer in any other organs, but there are no guarantees with cancer. They won't be able to know with certainty until I have surgery to remove the cancer and the lymph nodes are sent to pathology for testing. At this point, my head starts to spin and I feel like it might explode. *How can I be patient when so much is unknown?* There are no guaranteed marshmallows here – not even one!

☀ Devotional

Wait patiently on the Lord. – Psalm 27:14

Hebrews 6:13-15 says, *"When God made his promise to Abraham, since there was no one greater for him to swear by, he swore by himself, saying, 'I will surely bless you and give*

Day 3: Patience in Waiting

you many descendants.' And so after waiting patiently, Abraham received what was promised."

We know the end of the story, but we also know that before the promise was fulfilled, Abraham and Sarah made the mistake of running ahead of God, trying to figure out how to produce an heir using their own method. The result of their haste was an illegitimate heir, Ishmael, whom God could not bless in the way He had promised.

It's hard to wait when all you want is to get in there and fix things yourself and do things your way. It is important to remember the problem is not ours to fix – even though it feels that way! It's our job to surrender to God and allow His gracious love to guide us. As we wait for His complete and miraculous healing, we need to ask for patience without angst, fear, or discouragement. This will lead us to His perfect blessing in His perfect way. Whether it unfolds quickly or slowly, He has already provided for the outcome. He's doing His work – somewhere between.

Somewhere Between

God can, God can

And God will, God will

He'll fix it (God will fix it for you)

In the words of Dottie Peoples, God can. When you get to be my age, you don't always remember where you heard about things, but the good ideas stick with you. Somewhere along the line, I heard about something called a "God Can." It works like this: if you're waiting for or praying about something that is causing you to feel negative emotions, write it down on a piece of paper and literally put it into a can labeled "God." By doing this, you're releasing it to the care of God. The act of doing this reminds me of my mortal inability to force solutions or fix things according to my own agenda. I may not be patient enough to wait on my own, but God is not in a hurry. He can and will work things out in His time. Try it and see what you think!

Day 3: Patience in Waiting

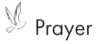 **Prayer**

Father, You know my heart. You know the waiting and the wondering are not comfortable for me. The days of uncertainty and questions sometimes lead me to places of discouragement, anxiety, anger, and distancing from You. Help me to remember, Lord, that You will not withhold any good thing from me. When I am waiting, it is because You know the perfect timing for bringing things together for my good. You know how my story is written. Be patient with me as I learn to love You more, and trust in Your sovereignty in all circumstances. I pray this in Jesus' name, Amen.

∽ DAY 4 ∽

Listening for the Holy Spirit's Voice

I don't know about you, but as a kid, I lived for roller coasters. Exciting, scream-worthy, and made me feel like I could fly, yet I still felt safe and protected. They left me feeling exhilarated! But then, I tried recapturing this same feeling in my forties – ha! My head kept saying "Maybe you should reconsider…", but the child in my heart was screaming "Go for it!" Well, let me tell you, there was no exhilaration all those decades later – just nauseating dizziness. I should have listened to my brain!

⚘ My Journey

Searching for answers, treatment options, and hope, our cancer-coaster ride has been less than stellar. We met with a

Day 4: Listening for the Holy Spirit's Voice

surgeon who made recommendations we weren't too comfortable with. We prayed about it, listened to the nudging of the Holy Spirit and decided to get a second opinion. We were told that our choices were limited because of insurance, but even that didn't have us throwing in the towel. We prayed again and again for divine favor and intervention. Miraculously, our agent got us switched to a company that allowed us to go to the Rogel Cancer Center at the University of Michigan to get that much-needed second opinion. *Praise the Lord! Thank you, Lord! What a big win.* Even when life seems bleak, God is working behind the scenes to make the impossible possible. I was so glad we listened to our Spirit nudge and pressed in!

When you drive, does your mind wander? Not mine! Drive times are when God speaks to me most clearly and has my undivided attention. As I was driving a route I know very well, I heard the Lord give me some direction on how I was to deal with my words and thoughts about cancer: *Whenever you read the Word and it mentions Satan, the enemy, or anything that refers to the demonic, substitute it with the word "cancer."*

When you need to speak the word "cancer," declare my name. I am above all diseases, cancer included.

The ~~thief~~ Cancer comes to steal, kill and destroy, but I have come that they might have life, and have it to the full. – John 10:10

Wow! This made so much sense to me because Jesus did come to defeat the enemy of our souls. I am so grateful for the leading of the Holy Spirit and His peace woven into every step of this journey.

☀ Devotional

People of Zion, who live in Jerusalem, you will weep no more. How gracious he will be when you cry for help! As soon as he hears, he will answer you. Though the Lord gives you the bread of adversity and the water of affliction, your teachers will be hidden no more; with your own eyes you will see them. Whether you turn to the right or to the left, your ears will hear

Day 4: Listening for the Holy Spirit's Voice

a voice behind you saying, "This is the way; walk in it." – Isaiah 30:19-21

Listening has become somewhat of a lost art. We can find ourselves so busy that we fail to stop and listen to what the Holy Spirit is saying to us. If we are to hear Him clearly, we need to create time in spaces where He deservedly has our undivided attention. If cancer comes to kill, steal and destroy, then the last thing Satan wants is for us to hear God's truth, let alone be in a space to listen for it. God wants us to thrive, not just survive. Jesus wants to speak truth loudly into our ears about who He is and who we are in Him. He wants to drown out the whispers and lies of the enemy that say we don't have choices and are doomed to eternal death. Today, we close our ears to the enemy and decide to actively listen for the voice of the Holy Spirit, walking boldly in the truth of what we hear. Satan will have to flee!

Find a quiet place to get alone with God. Sit in stillness and take time to listen for the voice of the Holy Spirit. Write down any verse, phrase, image, or song He brings to your mind, and ask Him to give you an understanding of what that means for you in this journey. You may never have done this before, but that's okay! Give it a try because you might just be surprised at how and what He speaks to you as you listen.

Prayer

Holy Spirit, I need You. I can get so distracted by worldly things and sometimes fail to quiet my heart and be still before You. Give me direction about what I should do or which way I should go. Help me to follow Your lead, even if it seems unorthodox, scary, or different from what I expect. Make Your voice so loud and clear that I can't miss what You are speaking to me. Guide me in truth and let Your peace abide in my heart as I faithfully follow. In Jesus' name I pray, Amen.

ᴄᴏ DAY 5 ᴄᴏ

Sheltered in His Presence

I've always loved the Psalms because of how they express emotions – so real and tangibly raw. Even when the Psalmists lament the inevitable sorrows of life, by the end, they are declaring the highest praises remain for our magnificent, loving, and faithful God. They don't sugar coat our brokenness or the brokenness of our world, but anchor our hope in our faithful Father and the everlasting promise of His full redemption. Every time I open my Bible to Psalm 91, I am reminded that as I dwell in the presence of God, I will find protection, peace, and strength. Every day, no matter what comes my way!

⚘ My Journey

I came to truly know Jesus about twenty-five years ago when I was around the age of 36. I have one of those forever friends

— you know, the ones that maybe you don't see all the time, but when you do, it's like no time has passed. I would call her my soul sister, and she is one of the reasons why I came to know Jesus. Our friendship is deeply rooted in our mutual faith. Whenever we get the opportunity (which isn't as often as we'd like these days), we get out on Goguac Lake to kayak, then have a bite to eat and fellowship. My cup is always overflowing after an evening with Becky, and I'm so lucky to have a friend like her in my life. Recently, during one of our get-togethers, we crafted a beautiful pink cancer ribbon blanket. It's almost an exact replica of one I made for a friend years ago when she was diagnosed with breast cancer. Back then, I never would have imagined that one day I would be making another one for my own cancer journey.

In the first year of dating my now husband, Dave, he gifted me a pink panda bear. If you squeeze its chest, you can feel its heartbeat. Truth be told, I loved this silly little bear. While a bit juvenile for a grown woman, it was so sweet because it came from Dave, someone who unconditionally and endlessly loved me, and wasn't afraid to show it! Today, I have this bear

Day 5: Sheltered in His Presence

alongside my new pink blanket – they match perfectly! – and they both bring me feelings of comfort and peace. I can hear God saying "I'm providing for you and protecting you through those closest to you and the many, many others who will love and help you along the way. Continue to dwell in Me and I will cover you. I will provide refuge and peace." Who would've thought a blanket and pink panda bear could mean so much? Man, God is good!

Devotional

Whoever dwells in the shelter of the Most High
*   will rest in the shadow of the Almighty.*
I will say of the Lord, "He is my refuge and my fortress,
*   my God, in whom I trust."*
Surely he will save you
*   from the fowler's snare*
*   and from the deadly pestilence.*
He will cover you with his feathers,
*   and under his wings you will find refuge;*
*   his faithfulness will be your shield and rampart.*

Somewhere Between

You will not fear the terror of night,
  nor the arrow that flies by day,
nor the pestilence that stalks in the darkness,
  nor the plague that destroys at midday.
A thousand may fall at your side,
  ten thousand at your right hand,
  but it will not come near you.
You will only observe with your eyes
  and see the punishment of the wicked.
If you say, "The Lord is my refuge,"
  and you make the Most High your dwelling,
no harm will overtake you,
  no disaster will come near your tent.
For he will command his angels concerning you
  to guard you in all your ways;
they will lift you up in their hands,
  so that you will not strike your foot against a stone.
You will tread on the lion and the cobra;
  you will trample the great lion and the serpent.
"Because he loves me," says the Lord, "I will rescue him;
  I will protect him, for he acknowledges my name.

Day 5: Sheltered in His Presence

He will call on me, and I will answer him;
  I will be with him in trouble,
  I will deliver him and honor him.
With long life I will satisfy him
  and show him my salvation." – Psalm 91

Find a blanket, a photo, or something of meaning that brings you comfort and helps you remember that God is your ever-present help in times of trouble. You are safe with Him always.

Prayer

Hear my prayer, O Lord. My heart is fixed on You. I am thankful that when I come to You with my emotions, You understand the deep places within me even before I say a word. I am grateful to You, Lord, for Your promise to be my fortress, to protect, rescue, and deliver me as I honor and acknowledge Your name. Thank You for loving me, saving me from every disaster, and being such a faithful friend. Continue to cover me with Your love and keep me close to Your heart. In Jesus' name I pray, Amen.

~ DAY 6 ~

Old Command, New Ink

Not all that long ago, people with tattoos were thought of in a very negative light. Men with tattoos were assumed to be criminals, gang members, bikers, or perhaps military men. Today, tattoos have become very popular with people in nearly every walk of life. The designs are creative and can be used to express the thoughts and emotions of their wearers. Tattoos may even be a reminder of something impactful in that person's life. Some tattoos are barely noticeable, while others are full sleeves of colorful images that cover every square inch of an arm. Whether it's a cartoon character, a butterfly, or a beautiful cross, a tattoo is a personal statement etched in skin.

Somewhere Between

🎗 My Journey

After our first meeting with my team at the Cancer Center, my doctors reviewed all the diagnostic tests and concluded that due to the size and position of the tumor, there was no way to save my breast. Meaning, a mastectomy was the only option. Hearing this news left me feeling raw and fragile. I needed to encourage myself for what I knew would be a serious challenge. Before my first surgery, I decided to get a tattoo. I know that might not be for everyone, but for me it was a personal statement of faith. I found a local, reputable shop and went in to get a few pretty flowers and the words from Joshua 1:9 inked onto my forearm. I wanted to be able to easily remember what God had commanded Joshua:

Be strong and courageous. Do not be afraid; do not be discouraged, for the Lord your God will be with you wherever you go.

The only reason I can be strong and courageous in the face of this illness is because of my faith in Jesus. He knows what is

Day 6: Old Command, New Ink

ahead because He wrote my story. So even now, when I look at the three delicate flowers adorning the scripture verse on my arm, I can feel His presence, encouraging me to fight the good fight. I read the words and am reminded that He's in control.

You may not be someone who would ever get a tattoo, but you can find your own way to encourage yourself. Write a verse on a sticky note and leave it on your bathroom mirror for a daily reminder from the beginning every day. Find stillness and meditate on some of your favorite encouraging verses and declare them over yourself. Make a vision board of all the things you want to do during or after your treatment is over and place it somewhere you will see often. You are blessed and highly favored, cancer or not, so eyes up, child of the Most High God! You're going to get there!

Devotional

The path to our Promised Land of healing is at times overwhelming. There will be days we will have dips in our faith, trust, and positive outlook for the future. We may fail to stay as close to Him as we want. Even so, the first chapter of Joshua reminds us to be careful to obey God's word, keeping it on our lips. It tells us not to turn to the right or to the left, but to meditate on it day and night, so that we may be careful to do everything written in it. Then we will be successful and prosper wherever we go. We know the promises of God are waiting for us if we will line up with what we already know about God's faithful character and good purpose for our lives. Do we know exactly what that will look like? No, but we can be strong in the Lord and the power of His might. Declare it today! We will be courageous in our actions because His Spirit lives in us and will be with us wherever we go. And we will reach that promised land. He will reveal it to us step by step as we stay close to Him. Of this, we can be sure!

 Prayer

Father, thank You that doctors and medical professionals have been given wisdom to help me understand the issues and give direction for addressing them. Thank You for encouraging my

Day 6: Old Command, New Ink

heart as I face the many battles ahead. Thank You, too, that I can trust that You are always in control and will lead me in the path You know is best for me. When I feel raw and fragile, I am so grateful I can always count on You to be my comfort, strength, and peace. Help me not to worry about the journey but to simply follow Your direction. I pray this all in Jesus' name, Amen.

DAY 7

Never Alone

Some people are extreme extroverts, those who feel energized and in their "element" with others or in a large group. However, that's not me. I value my alone time. Before I married Dave, I spent a lot of years being single and I grew comfortable being alone. When I'm with people, I'm fully present and enjoy being part of a community, but I have a need to spend time alone, too. Whether you're an introvert or extrovert, I want to remind you that we are never truly alone. Even when we are physically alone, God is always with us.

My Journey

It was time to get a CT scan for a better picture of the exact size of the tumor and its specific placement. At my appointment, I put on headphones and played soft music to help me relax and remain still during the process. I softly hummed as I went into

Day 7: Never Alone

the tube. I was calm because my family and I had been praying for and fully expecting God to perform a miracle. We prayed that the three-centimeter tumor would completely disappear. I imagined that we'd get halfway through the imaging and stop because they couldn't find anything. I must admit, I was more than a little disappointed when the scan continued as normal.

As I lay there, face-down, head-first in the cold tube, I was physically alone but I never really felt alone. I could feel the presence of the Holy Spirit hovering over me and giving me peace. There was no worry or fear. I knew I was surrounded by the presence of God, loved and supported by Dave, my family, and friends. While the appointment didn't abruptly stop in the middle to announce a miracle, I experienced my own miracle with this overwhelming peace and positivity.

Just before I came out of the tube, I heard the melody and powerful lyrics of Kari Jobe's, *I Am Not Alone.* Our God is amazing, even in the little details of our lives.

When I walk through deep waters
I know that You will be with me
When I'm standing in the fire
I will not be overcome
Through the valley of the shadow
I will not fear
I am not alone
I am not alone
You will go before me
You will never leave me – Kari Jobe, I Am Not Alone

☀ Devotional

In the book of Exodus, we read about the Israelites escaping Egypt and heading toward their Promised Land. They were going in blind and not doing very well trusting God or their leader, Moses. Think of how alone he must've felt! But God did not leave Moses to his own devices. He provided His presence in the form of a pillar of cloud by day and a pillar of fire by night to lead His people in the way that they should go. This was God's miraculous provision for them and the fulfillment of

Day 7: Never Alone

His promise to never leave or forsake them. He was faithful to His word and His covenant with Israel even when Israel lacked faith. Likewise, God never leaves us alone to figure things out by ourselves. He gives us His Word and provides miraculous signposts to help us remember He is always with us; we are never alone. Look for the signposts God gives you to comfort, guide, and show you He's right there with you.

Prayer

Holy Spirit, I am amazed by You. I love You, and the intimate way You know me and know what I need at the exact moment I need it. You come into every one of my situations and minister to me in such specific and personal ways. Help me to look for You in the small things and realize that You are ever present with me, even when I don't know it or can't feel it. Give me Your presence and peace. In Jesus' name, Amen.

∽ DAY 8 ∾

Singing in the Storm

Worship is part of every human's DNA. God created us to fellowship with Him, to worship, and praise. Singing comes naturally to children and when they sing, it puts a smile on the faces of all those around them. There's something about singing that brings joy to both the singer and the Lord. Lyrics and melodies can touch a person's heart like nothing else can and our worship is the most authentic outpourings of our hearts to the heart of God.

♦ My Journey

Before I met Dave, one of the things I asked God for was a husband who would love to sing and worship as much as I did, so we could sing together. As usual, God didn't disappoint. Dave has the same worship DNA as I do. The only difference is that he has a much better voice than me! We spontaneously

Day 8: Singing in the Storm

sing together nearly every day, and it brings joy to my heart. The day we drove to the University of Michigan for a second opinion on my treatment strategy, we sang worship songs the entire time. It was a sacrifice of praise in the midst of our storm.

When we arrived, we immediately began appointments – six hours of back-to-back appointments, to be exact! We met with experts in radiology, consulted with the tumor board, various surgeons, and a breast reconstructive specialist. Each person we met was helpful, positive, and professional with seamless transitions from one specialist to another. They took as much time as we needed to address every question and concern we had. It felt like I was the only patient there.

After those six hours, we had a full plan of action in place. We reviewed all the testing, and the team didn't see the need for preemptive chemotherapy to shrink the tumor. They were confident that a mastectomy would be sufficient to eradicate the cancer. If my lymph nodes were clear, I might be able to have surgery, start reconstruction and be on my way without any chemotherapy or radiation. I can't tell you how joyful this possibility made us! While this plan still involved a mastectomy and clear lymph nodes were not a guarantee, I fully leaned into the idea and belief that God was going to stop this invasion and keep it from spreading further. Short of the complete and total miraculous healing we had been feverishly praying for, this was the next best scenario. Dave and I rejoiced together all the way home – and sang more!

☀ Devotional

How we respond to a battle, or a storm makes all the difference!

In II Chronicles 20, we read about King Jehoshaphat's impending battle with the foreign nations of the surrounding territories. These enemies were planning a concerted attack on Israel to take the land the Lord had given them in His covenant with Abraham. King Jehoshaphat and his troops were outnumbered on every side, but the Lord sent a prophet from among them to deliver God's message. The Lord told the

Day 8: Singing in the Storm

people to stand still and let Him fight for them because He would surely give them the victory.

On the day of battle, King Jehoshaphat sent out the worshipers in front of the troops. Their mouths were filled with praises to His name and holy splendor. When they began to sing, the Lord caused their enemies to turn on each other and destroy themselves. Israel never had to raise a sword and they plundered all the valuable weapons, clothing, and goods that were among the dead. The victory was in their praise and worship of their great and mighty Conqueror.

Find your own song of praise to God as He goes before you and fights on your behalf. Sing it loud and proud. It is a joyful noise to the Lord and music to His ears.

Prayer

Father, I am constantly amazed by You and how You orchestrate every detail of every situation for my good. It is with joy in my heart that I worship and praise You for who You are. You are worthy of all praise, whether I am facing a multitude of enemies or fear of the future. Thank You that I can stand still, and let You fight for me, providing strategies to face my storms. Thank You for Your care and extravagant provision. Help me keep my eyes and heart always worshiping You. I pray this in Jesus' name, Amen.

⌒ DAY 9 ⌒

A New Thing

New beginnings can be exciting, terrifying – or a combination of both! In order for something new to begin, something has to end. New beginnings can be the result of a conscious choice made, of someone else's choices that impact us, or those that are an act of nature, like a tsunami or a sudden, unexpected illness. New beginnings are filled with potential!

🎗 My Journey

One day, I got a call from the scheduler at the hospital. They had a surgical opening and said I could go in for my mastectomy eight days from now. Immediately, I was reminded of the fact that the number eight has biblical significance but couldn't remember exactly why. I said yes to the appointment then started my research. In biblical terms, the number eight means "a new beginning."

In eight days, I will most certainly have a new beginning. There will be the death and removal of the cancer in my breast, followed by the rebirth of a healthier me that is now cancer free! It will take time to work through the physical and emotional pain of loss. I will need to adjust to the new creation of an artificial expander that will reside in my chest instead of what's been natural to me since adolescence. To be honest, I'm not sure what this "new beginning" will look or feel like. I don't know of a way to prepare myself for the adjustment that will come with whatever continued treatment may be necessary. I've never been here before, but, thankfully, I know Jesus has. He goes before me and prepares the way. When it seems like the road is too dark or wet or stormy for me to see beyond, I can count on Him to hold me close and lead the way.

Day 9: A New Thing

✹ Devotional

But now thus says the Lord,
he who created you, O Jacob,
he who formed you, O Israel:
"Fear not, for I have redeemed you;
I have called you by name, you are mine.
When you pass through the waters, I will be with you;
and through the rivers, they shall not overwhelm you;
when you walk through fire you shall not be burned,
and the flame shall not consume you
For I am the Lord your God,
the Holy One of Israel, your Savior – Isaiah 43:1-3

Remember not the former things,
nor consider the things of old.
Behold, I am doing a new thing;
now it springs forth, do you not perceive it?
I will make a way in the wilderness
and rivers in the desert – Isaiah 43:18-19

Whether you choose it or not, you can face each ending with confidence that God's new beginnings are often blessings in disguise. Take time to look back on times when you thought an ending would be a bad thing and it turned out to be something incredible. God is in the business of surprising us when we least expect it!

 Prayer

Father, thank You for the encouragement in Your Word that gives me new beginnings, a way in the wilderness, and streams in the desert. There's no way for me to embrace the unknown except to call on You and to fall into Your loving arms. Help me, Lord, to not see an ending, but a beginning You have prepared for me. I trust You, Lord, and count on Your faithfulness to fix the faulty picture in my life. Thank You for Your goodness, Lord, and for being ever present as You do a new thing in and through me. I pray this in Jesus' name, Amen.

DAY 10

Suspect Faith

We've all heard about people who say they have miraculous, supernatural powers. They say a God-given gift allows them to pray over people or lay hands on them and suddenly, those who were sick are miraculously healed. Some of these "healers" say they have lengthened legs, restored hearing to the deaf and sight to the blind, prayed babies into the wombs of infertile couples – the claims go on and on. We've come to find out that some of these "miracle workers" are nothing more than frauds. There are others however, who indeed seem to possess these healing gifts. The circumstances surrounding these events are often suspect and need to be verified in order to be believed; but I believe in miracles because I've experienced them.

Somewhere Between

🎗 My Journey

The clock is ticking down. Three days from now, I am scheduled to lose a body part. That's my immediate reality, but I haven't stopped praying for a miracle. Ridiculous faith like mine is always suspect and extreme to most people. When I tell people Jesus is going to heal me, many are dismissive or just plain sarcastic. I can't tell you how many professionals rolled their eyes or patronized me by saying things like, "Yeah, you just keep praying, honey," or "I guess it can't hurt if that helps you." I want so badly for them to see the power of God to really heal.

It hurts my heart that they are not open to the miraculous. It also hurts my heart that it hasn't happened yet. I know God can heal me completely and I don't know why He hasn't chosen to do so. Even so, I'm a lot like other biblical characters who were willing to believe miracles are possible even when the situational evidence didn't support the expectation. I am willing to look like a fool and risk being mocked in order to believe in the One who has the power to create the world, heal the sick,

Day 10: Suspect Faith

call the dead to life, and to raise Himself from the dead. If that sounds radical and extreme, that's because it is! Jesus is a completely different God who up-ends our paradigms and dismantles our traditions. Doctors follow scientifically-supported data points and studies, leaving little room for the miraculous. Believe me, I get it. Medical treatment does help cure many ailments and diseases, but it can't fix everything or explain a miracle when it does happen.

Will there be a last-minute miracle healing, a "Hail Mary" rescue with seconds to go in the game? I don't know. That's up to Jesus. He calls the shots in my life. Either way, in life or death, I will get healing. Whether that's with modern medical technology, the skill of surgeons and oncologists, a divine miracle, or because my days here are complete, I will be healed in Jesus' name! I won't give up on my first line of treatment. My great physician, Jesus Christ!

✺ Devotional

Again he entered the synagogue, and a man was there with a withered hand. And they watched Jesus, to see whether he would heal him on the Sabbath, so that they might accuse him. And he said to the man with the withered hand, "Come here." And he said to them, "Is it lawful on the Sabbath to do good or to do harm, to save life or to kill?" But they were silent. And he looked around at them with anger, grieved at their hardness of heart, and said to the man, "Stretch out your hand." He stretched it out, and his hand was restored. The Pharisees went out and immediately held counsel with the Herodians against him, how to destroy him. – Mark 3:1-6

The man's hand was useless to him, unable to function the way it was designed. I am sure he had grown used to this dysfunction and had adjusted to his circumstances. For this man to reach out and allow Jesus to touch his withered hand was probably exciting and intimidating. It meant exposing his shame for all to see. What if Jesus didn't really have the power to heal it? What if he took the risk and then it didn't happen?

Day 10: Suspect Faith

Would he be disappointed or feel stupid because he wanted something so badly? Would it be worth opening himself up to such public ridicule?

In the end, this man wanted healing more than he worried about what people would say or think. The idea that Jesus could and would heal anyone at any time was a threat to the religious authorities. It meant that He really was God and really could do things that would blow apart their traditions and paradigms. It's not unlike how the scientific world thinks about miracles today.

Maybe you've had the same questions as the man with the withered hand. I know I have. What do we do if Jesus doesn't heal us miraculously? Does it mean He can't, He won't, or doesn't care to? I encourage you to go to the Lord with your questions, anger, doubts, or fears. You're not alone in this. Pour it all out before Him and let Him speak to your heart. He is there to listen, and He hears you.

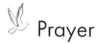 **Prayer**

Jesus, I remember the gospel stories that tell how You went from town to town, proclaiming the good news of the Kingdom and healing the sick. I know You are the same yesterday, today and forever, so I am confident You are able to supernaturally heal any diseases, and demonstrate Your power over all kinds of sickness. Help me to be willing to hold onto radical faith and leave the way of healing up to You. Thank You for listening when I come to You with my questions, fears, and doubts. Help me hear You in my struggles. I pray in Your name, Amen.

DAY 11

Levity Before Surgery

Have you ever thought about the fact that comedians are literally paid to make us laugh? They find the absurd, controversial, or irreverent inconsistencies in life and twist it into comical stories that leave us in stitches. A good joke or a funny movie has a special way of lifting my spirits, even on my worst days. I can recall times that I have laughed so hard, it was difficult to breathe. That's not particularly good for someone with asthma, but I'd rather laugh myself silly than be depressed over the seriousness of life. Laughter is really, good medicine!

My Journey

Those who know me best would tell you that I'm a realist and not particularly tactful or overly sensitive. I make light of a lot of things, even when they're serious. Cutting through the nonsense isn't always comfortable for everyone, but with me, "what you see is what you get." While my faith runs very deep, my unique sense of humor is also a big part of who I am and you'll either love it or wish I would keep it to myself! Dave is a jokester as well, so even whilst dealing with this very serious disease, we were able to have some laughs. If you can't stare a potentially life-threatening situation in the face and laugh at it, then you will probably find yourself wrapped up in fear, hopelessness, and depression. Since I hope never to be fearful, hopeless, or depressed, I make a point to constantly find ways to humor myself and others. Dave and I are similar in this way. We joke about getting a perky new set of boobs out of the deal. Maybe even a bit of liposuction on the side? Dave often asks me, "How is lefty today?" To which I respond, "Lefty is not right!" Alright, I know, it's not a side splitter, but good enough to land a smirk on our faces. We both know that laughter is good for the soul!

☀ Devotional

In Ecclesiastes 3:4, the Bible says there is a time to weep and a time to laugh.

Day 11: Levity Before Surgery

Cancer can bring us into times of emotional distress. No one can deny how hard cancer is and just as there are times to weep, we must also find time for laughter.

In John 10:10, Jesus said that *the thief (cancer) comes to kill, steal, and destroy, but He has come to give us life, and life to the full.* To me, abundant life means a life that includes plenty of laughter, even in difficult times.

A cheerful heart is good medicine, but a broken spirit saps a person's strength. — Proverbs 17:22

Sometimes the best way to face adversity and get to the other side is with a joke and a cheerful attitude. We're not going to change anything with a sour disposition, so we might as well try to find the silver lining in the cloud. Who knows? We might even find ourselves making God smile in the process!

Do something just for fun today, something that will make you laugh and bring joy to your soul.

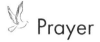 Prayer

Father, having cancer is a serious thing. At times, it consumes my thoughts and is a thief of joy. I thank You for the gift of laughter, for the things I can find humorous and the situations that tickle me. Help me to see how much You love watching me have childlike joy with even the smallest things. Keep me searching for the moments that make life enjoyable in every season. I pray this in Jesus' name, Amen.

∽ DAY 12 ∽

Deconstruction

Children are innately creative and their imaginations run wild. My grandchildren can spend hours using their creative energy with Legos. Every time they pull them out, they build the most innovative designs and colorful creations! Legos are designed to encourage creativity and can be configured and reconfigured in as many ways as a child can imagine. Build it, take it apart, build something new — the cycle is endless! Naturally, creatives aren't often boxed into doing things exactly the same way every time. New structures don't have to be perfect. It's more important that they are enjoyed. If you don't like what you've created, you can take it apart and make something new.

Somewhere Between

⚘ My Journey

Unlike all the choices you have in configuring Legos, Dave and I didn't have a lot of surgical options. The only real choice for dealing with my diagnosis was for doctors to physically deconstruct my breast with a mastectomy. I was given the option of reconstruction during the surgery, afterward, or not at all. Initially, I was unsure. The word "reconstruction" brought to mind visions of rebuilding something that would not feel natural to me. The doctors could replicate my breast, but never duplicate what was originally there. I was presented with a dizzying array of options for how this could be done. But, to be honest, it felt like I was picking out the make, model, and package available for a custom car. There would be risks involved and additional surgeries associated with matching my other breast. There would be pain associated with stretching skin and no guarantee that infection, radiation, or other issues wouldn't cause the process to fail. I started doubting if it was necessary. *How important is this to me? Is reconstruction worth*

Day 12: Deconstruction

the pain of the process with no guarantees of success? What do I have to gain and what do I have to lose?

After a lot of thought, Dave and I decided the easiest and least disruptive option would be to have immediate reconstruction with an implant. Instead of waking up with a flat chest, I would wake up with a soft plastic expander where my breast used to be, and we would start the process of expansion. If you are going through a similar decision, I encourage you to ask yourself the same questions I did and make a decision that is right for you. There is no right or wrong way!

❋ Devotional

Any time we have to make a hard decision, we assess the risk and reward. But we sometimes find ourselves in a situation with no clear cut answer. It feels like a toss-up that could go either way. At the same time, these big decisions often have long term consequences and can make us question what we believe about God, about His character, His goodness, and His plan for our lives.

Unless it's a salvation issue or a moral decision we must make, it's important to remember that we really can't make a wrong decision.

God works all things together for good for those who love Him and are called according to his purpose. — Romans 8:28

As we work through hard decisions, we can rest in His grace and make these decisions with confidence. There's grace in the gray.

Prayer

Father, I come to You with so many questions. There are times I have to make choices that I am unsure of or maybe even a little too overwhelmed to make. I need wisdom and direction from the Holy Spirit. I need to hear Your voice amidst the loudness of my options. Help me to consider all the facts but also what You speak to me in the still quiet moments of the morning or evening. Give me the mind of Christ and give me

Day 12: Deconstruction

grace in the process of making decisions. I pray in Jesus' name, Amen.

DAY 13

Loss and Wholeness

Author Shel Silverstein wrote a book in the 1980s called *The Missing Piece*. It is a story about a large round stone, which has lost part of itself and goes from place to place looking for the piece it has lost. The stone feels incomplete and rolls down the path looking for other stones that could complete it. The stone finds other pieces that have the potential to fit, but they are not perfect, so the stone keeps rolling along. Finally, the stone finds its missing piece. At first it seems like the perfect fit but in time the stone realizes the replacement is not the solution that it was thought to be. In the end, the stone decides it can still be happy and complete even if it is always missing a piece.

I wonder if I can ever feel the same about my missing breast?

Day 13: Loss and Wholeness

🎗 My Journey

Before I was wheeled into the operating room, Dave prayed over me, kissed me, and with a wave goodbye, I was off. I thought I was prepared for what was ahead. It's kind of like when a woman gives birth to her first baby. If she's anything like me, she actually has no idea what is about to happen. Waking up after surgery, I felt no pain at all. I could see a small drain tube coming from my underarm and a noticeable bump under layers of bandages on my chest. That bump told me that the surgery was over and the expander was in.

Dave didn't care if I would have a breast or not and didn't really think it was necessary. I even questioned it, but for me, it came down to the idea of being made whole again. When you feel loss, you know what's missing and you desperately want to get it back. Losing something that's a part of you feels awful. You wonder how you will ever feel or look like you again. But, the fact is that you won't. No matter how much time, money, or energy you spend to rebuild or restore something you've lost, it's never going to be the same. You are forever changed.

Change is uncomfortable. It challenges you, stretches you, and at times you question whether or not it's worth it. There's no guarantee it will be better, or the end result will be what you hoped for. But you have to keep hanging onto hope.

☀ Devotional

Loss is a real thing and impacts all of us. It's part of the curse and our human condition that no one can escape. Whether it's the loss of a friend, family member, a job, dream, or even a body part, loss changes us. It stretches us physically, emotionally, and spiritually. It reminds us of all the losses we have experienced over the years and the ways we've been forced to change because of them. Before we can reconstruct our physical, mental, and spiritual selves to be pleasing to God, He gives us the opportunity to deconstruct all our faulty, diseased ideas about Him and His goodness. We have to offer

Day 13: Loss and Wholeness

ourselves completely to Him and challenge our worldly ways of thinking.

The times of deconstructing and rebuilding are never without risk or pain. It's uncomfortable. But God always walks those painful roads with us in our desire to be made whole and more like Him. He expands our faith as we trust Him. He knows the risk will be worth the reward as He stretches and reshapes us. Over time, the Holy Spirit slowly teaches us how to surrender our will to His. None of this is natural to us, but it is healthier and serves the purpose God intends for it to serve. Truth be told, He alone is our missing piece. Without this searching and surrendering process, we cannot be made whole.

Therefore, I urge you, brothers and sisters, in view of God's mercy, to offer your bodies as a living sacrifice, holy and pleasing to God—this is your true and proper worship. Do not conform to the pattern of this world, but be transformed by the renewing of your mind. Then you will be able to test and approve what God's will is—his good, pleasing and perfect will. — Romans 12:1-2

Somewhere Between

If you're feeling a little lost and worried about how you will ever feel like yourself again, join the club. You know you're missing a piece of your body, but no one else does. Ultimately, our job is to present our broken physical bodies, emotional, and spiritual selves to the Lord and allow Him to do what only He can. Yes, loss is real, but our restoration is promised.

Prayer

Father, I come to You with all of who I am, both the good and bad. I lay my pain and loss at Your feet. I can't always understand Your ways, but I trust that in every loss I experience, You have only allowed it to happen for a purpose. I know You see, know, and understand my pain because You Yourself are acquainted with the loss of Your only Son, Jesus, for a greater purpose. Help me to remember that You began a good work in me and will see it through until completion. In Jesus' name, Amen.

DAY 14

The Pitfall of Pride

Growing up, I learned that there were two kinds of pride, one good and one bad. The good kind was having a sense of accomplishment for achieving something difficult or doing things with excellence. The bad kind was a character flaw leading to a feeling or attitude of superiority. I sometimes had difficulty differentiating between the two because I was not only competitive and achieved a lot to be proud of, but also didn't like anyone telling me what to do or how to do it. I thought I was smart enough to figure things out on my own and didn't need help from anyone. Pride had me coming and going.

Somewhere Between

🎗 My Journey

The mastectomy is over and my recovery has begun. The tumor was removed and the affected areas have been cleansed of all residual microscopic cells. We are still praying we will not need any additional treatment like chemotherapy or radiation, but won't know until more tests come back in about a week. Even if more treatment is needed, we know His grace will be sufficient. Now it's time for me to rest and heal, a tough task for someone as stubborn, independent, and determined as me. While those traits are a great combination from a worldly perspective, the opposite could be said when you put on your spiritual glasses. No one knows this better than my husband who lives with my beastly pride and is often caught up in the struggle. After five days of resistance, Dave kindly suggested that I take a shower. I was anxious about getting the drain tube and incisions wet so I dug in my heels. He responded by making me a garbage bag covering for my chest. Pretty creative I must say, but, unfortunately, I still found a way to criticize it. I wish I could blame it on the high dose of pain

Day 14: The Pitfall of Pride

medicine I was on, but anxiety crept in and made me a little more prickly than usual.

Admitting weakness and exposing vulnerabilities are not something I've done well. At this point, I want to be and do everything like I did before the surgery, even if I know it's not realistic. I was feeling really great for the first two days. No one, including the nurses, could believe how fast I was able to get up, move, eat a full meal, and smile like nothing had happened. I must admit I was feeling a little bit cocky about my progress. You know the overachiever in me was hoping to be the first fairly pain-free mastectomy patient on record. Well, you know what they say. Proverbs 16:18 reads, *"Pride goeth before destruction, and a haughty spirit before a fall."* Yep, you saw it coming — day three was a disaster!

It started with a terrible headache, chills, and nausea. I thought maybe I just had a bad migraine, so I took my medicine. About twelve hours later, I was hunched over the toilet, feeling like death warmed over. *It's probably these doggone narcotics I'm taking! I guess I could just stop taking them.* How do you decide between pain and puking? Not an easy choice, but the correct one. Now twelve hours later, that poison is out of my body and I am feeling better. Sounds like Tylenol is the best it's going to get for relieving my pain.

I'm a pretty tough cookie by most standards, but I guess it's time to boast about my weakness. My body is weak, but God is strong. I know I have to depend on His strength, even when I feel resistance. It's the story of the human condition, both physically and spiritually. I'm not sure I'll ever delight in my weakness, but I'm thankful for everyone who bears with me as I recover. I'm not ungrateful or unappreciative even when I seem to be. I'm just learning how to receive love and help graciously.

☀ Devotional

God's Kingdom economy is not like the economy of this world. Jesus says in order to gain life you must lose it and in order to be first you must be last. In order to be great, you must be a servant to all. In order to be strong, you must be weak.

Day 14: The Pitfall of Pride

Therefore, in order to keep me from becoming conceited, I was given a thorn in my flesh, a messenger of Satan, to torment me. Three times I pleaded with the Lord to take it away from me. But he said to me, "My grace is sufficient for you, for my power is made perfect in weakness." Therefore, I will boast all the more gladly about my weaknesses, so that Christ's power may rest on me. That is why, for Christ's sake, I delight in weaknesses, in insults, in hardships, in persecutions, in difficulties. For when I am weak, then I am strong. — II Corinthians 12:7-10

Like Paul, we all plead for this disease, this messenger of Satan to be taken from us in a miraculous way. However, more often than not, it still comes down to a surgery. We are forced to give up our pride and let others help us in our healing. It's important for us to examine how our pride has kept us from being a gracious recipient of other's grace. It's not easy to admit, but it's a necessary part of our physical healing and spiritual growth.

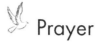 Prayer

Father, I am full of human pride. I often look to my own skills, stamina, and resources first instead of looking to You for help. I don't want to admit I am weak — or worse yet, I don't believe that I am. Help me, Lord, to be humble enough to realize I am merely human, broken in more places than just my physical body. Help me to see weakness as an opportunity to embrace Your sufficiency and the love of others. Make me appreciative and not too stubborn to accept help. I pray in Jesus' name, Amen.

⌒ DAY 15 ⌒

For Better or Worse

When little girls play dress up, it's a fun game of make believe. Inevitably, there comes a time when they've watched Cinderella enough times that they imagine themselves as the blushing bride marrying the handsome prince. They embrace the idea that finding and marrying their Prince Charming will be the ticket to a trouble-free life. Happily ever after! To all those little girls, I'd say that we need to rethink the idea that another person can make us happy or complete. The truth is that only a relationship with Jesus can do that.

🎗 My Journey

Not long after my diagnosis, I began to feel increasingly resentful. *This is so unfair! Dave and I have only been married for two years. We shouldn't have to deal with this!* I had the faulty idea we had already paid our dues in life, served God with great sacrifice, and somehow deserved to stroll into our golden years without any issues. I thought we were entitled to our very own happily ever after. I even confessed to one of my friends that I felt Dave had gotten a raw deal when he married me. I truly felt I had let him down by getting cancer— as if I had any control over it! My wise friend reminded me that no one knows what life will bring. When we sign up for marriage, we give God many opportunities to shape and mold us to be more like Jesus. Dave did not get a raw deal; we were gifted an opportunity to grow together through adversity and depend on God to see us through to the other side. I'm so grateful for the wisdom of friends!

I was recently scrolling through some of my writings and came across a note written in December 2019. It was a great reminder of all the things marriage is and why being married to the right person is so important. When I met Dave, I found a man who really showed me what authentic, faithful, and godly love was. Even in the most challenging situations, I know I can count on him to be that same guy.

Day 15: For Better or Worse

To my Dave, I dedicate this entry to you. I couldn't (and wouldn't want to) do this without you.

☀ Devotional

Most girls in my generation grew up believing that getting a ring and a husband would mean getting the life you always dreamed of. Saying "I do!" meant happiness and true love would make marriage effortless. You probably know that life isn't a fairytale, so where did that story come from? Let's see what saying "I do" from a biblical perspective means.

1.   You get to spend the rest of your life with someone who is as committed to you as you are to them. Even when you're a pain or they're a pain and you want them to go away, they won't. It's refusing to quit and working toward being so united there's no way on earth to separate your souls. "Until death do us part."

2.   It means you can do the things you love with them, but also doing things you never dreamed you'd have to do. As we

age, we have to take care of each other and it isn't always easy. Who wants to do all that's necessary when someone has a chronic illness like cancer, or has been disabled in an accident? Just taking care of someone with a nasty virus can be challenging, but that's exactly what married people say they'll do. "In sickness and in health."

3. It means being vulnerable and giving your spouse the power to call out your weaknesses, believing they will see the best in you even though it's not easy to see. It's learning to make adjustments as you share your time and personal space. It's learning to listen with an open mind when you'd rather just keep doing things the way you've always done them. It's encouraging your spouse when they're down, giving when you want to take, and forgiving when you're still angry. It's laughing until you think you're going to throw up and rejoicing when they succeed. "For better or worse."

4. It means being grateful for whatever you have, learning what is necessary and what is a luxury. It's about when to say "yes" and when to say, "no or not yet," so both of you can feel

Day 15: For Better or Worse

comfortable. It's about honoring the tithe for the sake of the Kingdom and using money for the benefit of others. "For richer or poorer."

5. It means no other person, place or thing (except your love for God) will ever be put in a place or position higher than your spouse. As you avoid physical connections or soul ties to outside images or people, you keep your relationship physically, emotionally and spiritually your one and only treasure. "Keeping only unto thee."

That may seem like a lot, but saying, "I do!" with these things in mind says that you understand marriage is not for your happiness, but for your completion. It is a human representation of a godly ideal. Real love is not only physical, emotional, and spiritual, but sacrificial and costly, too. It is worth everything it takes to get and keep the ring, the spouse, and the life you always dreamed of.

Take some time today to appreciate your spouse or significant others God has given you. Make a list of the things you appreciate about them and share it with them. Do something special to show them you care. They are as deeply affected as you are in this cancer journey, so try to remember that you're in this together.

Prayer

Father, I need You and I need others. You said it was not good for man to be alone, and You ordained marriage to be a physical representation of a spiritual reality. Thank You for my spouse, significant others, and all those who sacrifice their time and energy to pray with and for me . Thank You for those who care for me in good times and in difficulties. Help me remember that hardships are intended to help me grow in maturity and compassion for others. Help me appreciate these experiences as they serve to conform me more and more to the image of Christ. I pray this in Jesus' name, Amen.

∽ DAY 16 ∽

Fight My Battles

I really enjoy watching a good movie. My favorite genres are action, sci-fi, and an occasional comedy. My least favorite are horror, prison, and war movies. They all contain some kind of psychotic battle with mass carnage that leaves me feeling physically ill. Just like the endless Halloween movies, there's always a scene where the bad guy is killed and then miraculously sits up and continues terrorizing their victims. It's horrifying! I want the bad guys to be annihilated and gone for good. Maybe that's why I hate horror movies. The endings keep you hanging, wondering if it's a setup for a sequel of scariness.

℞ My Journey

After the initial surgery, Dave and I got the equivalent of a horror movie call from the Cancer Center. The surgical team had removed everything they saw as a cancerous threat to my life, but when the pathology report came back, it indicated microscopic amounts of cancer were found in the Sentinel Lymph Node. This was not what we were expecting! Dave and I had already declared a complete victory, and this news had no place in my story. We thought the villain was dead, but it was still there, hiding in the shadows.

Microscopic amounts of cancer have the potential of spreading to other parts of the body and re-starting the entire battle again. This can happen weeks, months, or even years into the future. Cancer is a ruthless, brutal foe, attacking generations of families, and it does not give up until it totally annihilates its victim. I'm not going to lie — we were devastated! *What the heck happened? Didn't we pray and ask for divine healing? Why would God allow any cancer to stay in my body? If He loves me, where is He in all this and why isn't He protecting me?*

It's so disappointing to pray, do everything you know to do, and still not get the results you want. I know I'm not alone in feeling upset and angry, but honestly, I was just so sad and disappointed. I really did not understand.

Day 16: Fight My Battles

The new next steps include more appointments with my medical team to develop and decide on a new "battle plan." There's no defined strategy (yet) but I'm ready to fight this head on. We are determined: this next battle will win the war and completely obliterate the monster. It would be easy for us to feel defeat, but even in our deep disappointment, we are trusting in the Lord for a great and total victory. We fight our battles through praise as we make war on the floor in prayer.

Devotional

In I Kings 19, Elijah was fresh off a victory at Mount Carmel where he gained a great victory for the Lord. He had just humiliated and slaughtered 400 prophets of Baal for their idolatry and ended a drought over the land of Israel for three and a half years.

Elijah should have felt empowered and ready for the next battle. Instead, he ran away from the threats of wicked queen Jezebel and hid in a desert! What happened? Elijah had quickly forgotten how the Lord had given him victory and now he was having a pity party. He even asked God to let him die. Two different times, angels were sent from heaven to feed and minister to him. God didn't leave Elijah in a wilderness but led him to a place where He could speak to him.

God strengthened Elijah before confronting him by asking, "What are you doing here?" Had he forgotten his identity so quickly and his powerful God? Just look at what He had already done. Elijah thought he was alone, but he wasn't. The I Am was with him and so were thousands of others. He needed to get up and keep going!

Setbacks are a part of the cancer journey. As in many other areas of life, it's not always a straight line to victory. Every story has twists and turns. The ups and downs of life are distinct but not unique. There's nothing God doesn't understand and no amount of questioning or disappointment He can't handle. He ministers to us and never leaves us alone. Dancing with the Lord sometimes looks like a Tango and other times like a ChaCha. It may be one step forward and two steps back, but the experience is never wasted.

Day 16: Fight My Battles

Prayer

Father, I come to You with my disappointments and broken expectations. I have done everything I can to follow Your lead, yet there are still times when the enemy seems to be winning. I know You see the situation from beginning to end, so help me trust You no matter what the circumstances look like. You are fighting for me and surrounding me with Your protection. Help me do whatever You say, even when I don't understand. I pray this in Jesus' name, Amen.

∽ DAY 17 ∽

Beautiful in its Own Time

Fall is my favorite season. I love the crisp, not too cold air, the bonfire smell, and the taste of hot apple cider and doughnuts. I especially love the crackle of fallen leaves beneath my feet. I never tire of watching as the leaves turn from green to gorgeous reds, yellows, oranges, and browns. When I was a kid, I was fascinated with science and the process of things like photosynthesis and osmosis. *Yep, I'm nerdy like that!* I was mesmerized by the process of leaves changing from summer green to something completely different looking in the fall.

Imagine my shock when I discovered this transformation wasn't a magic trick of nature, but simply a lack of chlorophyll production that happens naturally every year before winter. The process was designed to reveal the leaves' true colors before they literally fell off the tree and died. While most girls

Day 17: Beautiful In Its Own Time

were busy playing with Barbie dolls or having tea parties, I was trying to figure out how the death of healthy leaves could create such delight and beauty for human eyes. I was totally unaware that these "behind the scenes" processes were going on in nature all the time. It simply never occurred to me. It's just how complex and cool God has designed our world. From the tiniest microscopic cells to the complexities of the solar system, our Creator put every system together and made each work in perfect harmony with the others. His timing in everything is perfect!

⸙ My Journey

After our follow up visit at the Cancer Center, we got more mixed news. The tumor had been successfully removed, but they were not able to get clear margins. I didn't know what that meant, but the doctor explained that a clear margin was at least two centimeters of healthy tissue between the site where the cancer was and the unaffected tissue. The surgeon was only able to get a margin of one centimeter because the tumor was very close to my chest wall. This meant if any cancer cells were left behind and able to push through, these cells would likely invade my chest wall, lungs, and other organs. If this happened, the cancer would be considered Stage 4 metastatic. The end of that journey would be the news that I could be treated and made comfortable, but not cured.

My medical team strongly suggested six weeks of daily radiation, a total of 30 rounds, hormone suppression therapy, and possibly chemotherapy as well. Dave and I talked extensively about chemotherapy and neither of us were interested in going that route. We asked for one more test called an Oncotype to give me a score to better determine if chemotherapy is absolutely necessary. It would take three weeks to get those results, so in the meantime, I planned to keep praying, working from home, and healing from surgery.

Day 17: Beautiful In Its Own Time

❋ Devotional

Ecclesiastes 3 is a beautifully written passage about the fact that there is a time and season for everything under Heaven. Dave and I have marveled at God's timing. There's no good time to get cancer, yet the changing of the leaves reminds us that for everything there is a season. Just as removing life-giving chlorophyll allows us to see the true colors of the leaves, removing all the "goodness of physical, financial, and emotional" blessings we take for granted reveals in us the true colors of who we really are.

Will we continue to believe in the goodness of God? Will we accept this mess as part of our story and God's bigger picture for the Kingdom? Or will our faith and spirits wither and die? We may be withering or feel like life itself is being sucked out of us, but we are still confident there is delight and beauty to behold in the process.

At the end of this famous passage, the author of Ecclesiastes says to be joyful and do good as long as we live. We should eat and drink and take pleasure in all of this toil — this is God's gift to us. Do just that and trust the Lord to make everything beautiful in its own time.

 Prayer

Father, I love You. Your timing is perfect and nothing happens until the fullness of Your timeframe is revealed. Where I see an ending, Lord, You see a beginning. You always have a behind the scenes plan to bring me joy if I look to You for insight into what is truly happening. I know that endings are necessary for new life to begin, so help me embrace Your timing and trust Your resurrection power. I pray in Jesus' name, Amen.

∽ DAY 18 ∽

No Worries

My grandma used to say, "little pitchers have big ears." I had no idea what that meant until I was older and my mom explained it to me. She said that the expression was used to warn someone that a child was in the room and the person speaking should be careful about what they were saying. My grandma was afraid the grandchildren would overhear an inappropriate conversation and repeat it. She also wanted to protect us from being exposed to inappropriate topics as a result of eavesdropping. You never can tell who is listening.

⚛ My Journey

One morning after breakfast, Dave and I were discussing all the emotions that go along with fighting cancer. We talked about how easy it is for worry, doubt, anger, and sadness to creep into our daily lives and make things that should be simple become very confusing and troublesome. We prayed together and asked the Lord to help us understand how these emotions were negatively impacting us and to come to terms with the discrepancies between what the Word says about miracles and healing and the reality of this ongoing illness.

The very next day, I received a package in the mail from an organization in Dallas, Texas. Enclosed were two books about cancer, a perfect pair: one was written by a pastor who had been healed from Stage IV Melanoma, and the other written by his wife who was his caregiver during this ordeal. They had written the books to help Christians deal with the exact questions that we had been asking about aligning our emotions with our faith. We were both blown away by the timing of this special delivery. These books had obviously been sent in the mail and were on the way to our home before we ever talked about it or prayed for answers!

Later in the day, I casually mentioned to Dave that it would be really nice if we had something other than water to drink —

Day 18: No Worries

maybe some cider! Within a couple of hours, one of our friends dropped off a meal and had stopped by a farm to pick up a gallon of apple cider. It was as if God Himself was eavesdropping in on our conversation. Imagine that! That's just who God is! He knows what we need before we even ask and makes sure we are provided for, even in the tiniest things like a beverage.

☀ Devotional

Therefore I tell you, do not be anxious about your life, what you will eat or what you will drink, nor about your body, what you will put on. Is not life more than food, and the body more than clothing? Look at the birds of the air: they neither sow nor reap nor gather into barns, and yet your heavenly Father feeds them. Are you not of more value than they? And which of you by being anxious can add a single hour to his span of life? And why are you anxious about clothing? Consider the lilies of the field, how they grow: they neither toil nor spin, yet I tell you, even Solomon in all his glory was not arrayed like one of these. But if God so clothes the grass of the field, which today is alive and tomorrow is thrown into the oven, will he not much more clothe you, O you of little faith? Therefore do not be anxious, saying, 'What shall we eat?' or 'What shall we drink?' or 'What shall we wear?' For the Gentiles seek after all these things, and your heavenly Father knows that you need them all. But seek first the kingdom of God and his righteousness, and all these things will be added to you. — Matthew 6:25-34

In this passage, Matthew recounts a scenario about Jesus taking care of the physical aspects of our lives. This can be worrisome when you're looking at managing meals, daily chores, or the financial responsibility of paying for medical treatment. Even more so, the same can be said about the emotional and spiritual aspects of dealing with this disease. God knows what we need before we even ask! Our job is to seek first the Kingdom of God and His righteousness, and the rest will follow.

When we're in right standing with Him, we won't need to worry because we will naturally learn to trust in His goodness. When He does give us unexpected provisions and surprises, He

Day 18: No Worries

delights in doing so. He just likes to make sure we remember that He's already on it.

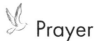 Prayer

Father, You are so good to me. You delight in reminding me of who You are and Your faithfulness to me. I can never fully understand how much You love and care for me, but I am so grateful that You do. Thank You for the big and small ways that You teach me to trust You, and surprise me with those things You know mean a lot to me. Help me to look for You to meet the needs in every area and situation. I pray in Jesus' name, Amen.

∽ DAY 19 ∽

Expanding

When my children were young, I hosted elaborate DIY birthday parties for them. I would use all my energy to blow up countless balloons, making the whole house feel colorful and festive. For someone with asthma like me, this was no easy task. I would blow a little bit at a time, rest between breaths and then blow some more. (Those magical balloon machines didn't exist back then!) It was a slow and methodical process, but one I eventually accomplished. It pushed my lung capacity to the limit, but I was determined to expand those balloons to get the party started.

☸ My Journey

During the first surgery to remove the cancer, I opted for immediate reconstruction. Now six weeks into recovery, my

Day 19: Expanding

incision is stable enough to start injecting saline into the implant port. The first time I remember hearing about the process was when I was lying on the examination table. Following a mastectomy, most women are numb in their breast area. I regained pretty much all my sensation in the area in a few weeks, so, unfortunately, I always felt the needles going into my skin as they filled the expander.

Every ten days, I would go to the office, have more saline added to the expander, and wait to see how it felt. *This is pretty cool! I can lose my boob and not only get something better in the process but get a lift on the right breast too! Score!* In my opinion this was a great consolation prize for enduring the loss.

Then I had to decide what size I wanted. *Well that's something new - a silver lining, for sure!* Not so fast, Lindy! Sadly, there was a lot more to the adjustment than I had expected. The stretching and pain of having a foreign object in my body was a challenge I had to press through to get to the other side. Who knew reconstruction would be so complicated?

✳ Devotional

Many women in the Bible were tested and stretched by God to see if they could be trusted with an expanded territory or a greater degree of influence. Some like Eve, Sarah, and Lot's wife failed their tests. They relied on their own understanding and ways to reach their own goals rather than following God's directions. By contrast, Hannah, Esther, and Mary, were all tested and were willing to go through the fire, to face pain, and adversity in order to achieve God's purpose for their lives.

We might think something will be easy, or at least, not that difficult, only to discover that it's far more challenging than we've been told. In these times of stretching, we must remember our physical, emotional, and spiritual growth are in process and we must rely on the Holy Spirit to grow in them. It's not going to happen overnight or be without sacrifice and pain. The more we submit ourselves to the work of the Spirit, the more He will empower us to become more like Jesus.

Day 19: Expanding

Setbacks and failures are to be expected, and the results will be worth far more than anything we will ever give up or lose along the way. This is where we experienced God's faithfulness. During times of testing, we take a breath, rest in the Lord, and trust Him to increase our strength and capacity with each new challenge. Each new level of expansion will bring us closer and closer to the goal set before us until it is finally accomplished.

Find time today to go back and look at how far you've come. There may be ways yet to go, but keep the momentum going! He is with you.

Prayer

Father, Your Word says I will have challenges in this life, but I should be of good cheer because You have overcome the world. Life is complicated. The stretching can feel too painful or like too much of a sacrifice for the end result. Help me, Lord, not to lean on my own understanding but to take time to listen to Your leading, rest in Your grace, and press through to the end. If this is the way You have planned for me to grow, I ask that You walk with me each step of the way. I pray this in Jesus' name, Amen.

DAY 20

Are You Willing?

I have always been quite adventurous and a little impulsive. If I see something that looks fun, I'm the first one to jump in — with both feet! I have a "you only live once" (YOLO!) kind of attitude. I mean, let's face it. I am the same woman who heard God calling me to mission work in China so I prepared myself, sold everything, left my family, and traveled across the globe to answer the call. It didn't matter that I didn't know Chinese, a single soul there, or had never even met a Chinese person! God said it, so I was doing it. This cancer journey was not that kind of adventure, though, and I was not anxious to embark on it.

My Journey

Dave and I have always agreed that we would avoid doing chemotherapy at any cost. We were open to considering radiation because it was a more targeted treatment approach. But chemotherapy? For us, it was a systemic "kill and destroy" method of treatment with both short- and long-term effects that we weren't willing to live with. We had watched others endure multiple rounds of chemotherapy with no improvements. For us, it was just too frightening to consider.

Fast forward and now chemotherapy and radiation were both on the table as viable paths forward. We were faced with the very thing we feared. The question became, "Are you willing to move forward in spite of your fear?" We were still waiting for my Oncotype test score which would determine whether or not chemotherapy would be effective. Since this Oncotype test was both sensitive and accurate, we weren't willing to commit to a chemotherapy plan without first knowing the results. We waited, prayed, and waited some more.

During this waiting period, I read an amazing book by Bob Sorge called *The Fire of Delayed Answers*. In it, Sorge explores the idea of suffering for a bigger purpose. We want our personal or spiritual development to be easy. We don't equate

Day 20: Are You Willing?

discipleship with sacrifice or suffering. Jesus, however, taught something completely different. He said we would have trouble in this world. Following Him would involve hardship and loss, even death, but the cost would be worth it. Jesus reassured His disciples that they need not be afraid because He had overcome the world and would be with them until the end of the age.

Throughout the weeks of waiting, I prayed I wouldn't have to endure the suffering I had seen others go through with chemotherapy. I prayed Dave and my family would not suffer watching me struggle to recover. I didn't want to develop a more "spiritual character" or suffer for some greater good. Amazingly during that time, the Holy Spirit was doing a tremendous work in my heart, too. I slowly stopped resisting the potential of pain and became willing to endure it — even embrace it — if that was required to make me more like Jesus. I felt my resistance begin to wane and a belief grew that He would be with me if my suffering was to be for a bigger purpose.

✸ Devotional

Digging deeper into the life and eventual death of Jesus shows us the perfect example of what it looks like to be a true disciple of Christ. Jesus was completely submissive to the will of the Father. In Matthew 26:39, Jesus was in the Garden of Gethsemane, praying to the Father. In His humanness, Jesus cried out, asking the Father to take the cup of crucifixion from Him. Yet Jesus was ultimately willing to do what was necessary for the Kingdom.

We can't compare our situation or suffering in any way to the agony that Jesus endured for our salvation. I am suggesting, however, the willingness to accept pain for a purpose is sometimes required of believers. It is through this purposeful pain that we become greater witnesses of His presence and faithfulness. It's something every disciple must wrestle with.

Where are you in the process? Are you willing?

Day 20: Are You Willing?

 Prayer

Father, You are the author and finisher of my faith. Without Your Spirit, faith would not even be possible. When I resist the idea of suffering, even if it's for a righteous cause, You are still able to soften my heart and make me willing to do things Your way. Help me daily to be willing to say, "Thy will be done." I pray in Jesus' name, Amen.

∽ DAY 21 ∾

Awareness

In the 1990s, something called Magic Eye became very popular. On the surface, it was 2D artwork that looked like a bunch of squiggles. If you held the picture really close to your face and slowly pulled it away, you would see a completely new 3D image hidden within the picture. Sounds cool, right? Okay, not super exciting if you compare it to the technology now at our fingertips, but it was revolutionary at the time. The thing is, not everybody could see the hidden 3D image. Only those who could focus their eyes could see it. The image inside the 2D picture didn't change. It was the focus of the viewer which made the difference.

⁂ My Journey

October is Breast Cancer Awareness Month, when you'll see ad after ad for testing to detect breast cancer and promoting

Day 21: Awareness

reminders for yearly mammograms. Of course, I did occasional self-exams and got yearly mammograms, but never in a million years did I think I would be the one in every eight women diagnosed with breast cancer. I had heard about 3D mammograms, but honestly, I didn't want to pay the extra money for one and didn't think it was necessary. Now I tell everyone that it's absolutely necessary! There are details a 2D mammogram cannot detect that are seen clearly with 3D technology.

My daughter is now aware of how crucial monthly self-exams are, especially now with a family history of breast cancer. Forget what insurance companies say about being forty before you qualify for a mammogram! She isn't 40 yet, but I insist that she gets one as an increasing number of women in their 20s and 30s are being diagnosed. Before my diagnosis, I was oblivious to what breast cancer was all about and ignorant about the early warning signs of cancer. I didn't have to be aware, or so I assumed. It had nothing to do with me...until it had everything to do with me.

My eyes are now drawn to pink ribbons on license plates, pink cancer t-shirts and other breast cancer symbols others overlook. Heck, I even bought a pink wig to wear in case I need to have chemo and lose all my hair. Funny how I overlooked it all, and never had an opinion about it until it was my battle. Being diagnosed with breast cancer has completely changed my perspective on just about everything.

I've had countless conversations with women I never knew had fought breast cancer and won. I didn't see it because they didn't lose their hair, didn't look sick, or didn't talk about it publicly. They only revealed it to those who had a similar focus. I have also had many conversations with people who have lost loved ones to this awful disease. Every person experiences it differently, and every story is unique. Being aware of these precious women and their families connects me to other cancer survivors and helps me to remember that Dave and I are not alone.

Day 21: Awareness

✸ Devotional

Cancer is a family affair; everyone is affected in different ways. It's also very personal for the person who is facing it. It's easy to get caught in the sadness of it all and the occasional pity party which we can fall into. We deal with the feeling we will always be broken. The truth is, we are forever altered and nothing we say or do will change that fact. But no matter how real those feelings may be (and I know how real they are!), we must never embrace sickness as our identity. As people, we tend to focus on the image and identity that is embedded in our 2D frame and miss the 3D reality of our wholeness in Christ. When we let the Word of God define who we are, we get the full picture and the assurance of Christ's redemption.

Since, then, you have been raised with Christ, set your hearts on things above, where Christ is, seated at the right hand of God. Set your minds on things above, not on earthly things. For you died, and your life is now hidden with Christ in God. When Christ, who is your life, appears, then you also will appear with him in glory. — Colossians 3:1-4

We set our focus on Him and what He says about us. The Bible says in I Peter 2:9: *"But you are a chosen people, a royal priesthood, a holy nation, God's special possession, that you may declare the praises of him who called you out of darkness into his wonderful light."* We may have cancer or may be a cancer overcomer, but we refuse to let malignancy define who we are. We are beloved daughters and sons of the King—cancer or not—and forever devoted followers of Jesus Christ. Let the image of Christ, and the confidence in His love and purpose for you be your focus.

Prayer

Father, I am fully aware of my brokenness and how cancer has impacted me and my family. But I do not embrace it as who I am. I only view myself in the light of who You are. If there is any identity that I choose to embrace, it is as a redeemed, restored child of the Most High God. I am one of those who claim You as Lord and Savior of my life. Help me to reject anything that

Day 21: Awareness

makes me feel inferior or less than who I am in You. I pray in Jesus' name, Amen.

DAY 22

Unending Praise

I was raised in the church. If the doors were open, my family was there. Even now, I remember nearly every word from every hymn I ever sang. When I found out I would be singing unending praises to Jesus in eternity, I was a little unnerved. I suppose I thought I would be singing those same hymns forever and ever and ever without an Amen. I didn't realize until much later, the way we demonstrate unending praises is as unique as we are. It may be in a song, poem, an artistic painting, or dance. Praise in whatever form is an offering of gratitude to God. We praise Him for who He is and what He has done. It is not an obligation but an honor to give Him our unending praise! I wish I would've known that as a teenager!

Day 22: Unending Praise

🎗 My Journey

Finally, the long awaited call: my phone rang and it was the oncologist calling to discuss my oncotype score. I quickly grabbed Dave and we braced ourselves for the worst, but also had peace about whatever we would hear. The news was far better than we had anticipated — she said that the score was relatively low. In fact, with an oncotype score as low as mine, there was no data that would suggest chemotherapy would be beneficial at all. We were ecstatic and shed tears of joy! I almost couldn't believe it. We continued to rejoice over this news with our families and friends for the next two days. I felt relieved, but also very satisfied. I finally passed this next test of my spiritual development and was willing to let my faith ride above my fear.

Devotional

Every day should be a time for praise to the Lord. But there are special times when we are exceedingly grateful for a specific blessing He has bestowed on us. These are times for exuberant praise!

I will extol the Lord at all times; his praise will always be on my lips.
I will glory in the Lord; let the afflicted hear and rejoice.
Glorify the Lord with me; let us exalt his name together.
I sought the Lord, and he answered me;
he delivered me from all my fears.
Those who look to him are radiant;
their faces are never covered with shame.
This poor man called, and the Lord heard him;
he saved him out of all his troubles.
The angel of the Lord encamps around those who fear him,
and he delivers them.
Taste and see that the Lord is good;
blessed is the one who takes refuge in him — Psalm 34:1-8

Day 22: Unending Praise

I encourage you to find time today and offer God your highest praise, no matter what your circumstances or where you are in your process. Whether it's a poem, song, dance, or something that is uniquely you — whatever that looks like — make it a sacrifice of unending praise. He inhabits the praises of His people!

Prayer

How can I not praise You for your ever-present Spirit and everlasting love? There are times when I doubt Your goodness and question Your plans, but then You remind me of Your faithfulness. Thank You for only giving me Your best. Thank You for Your grace and mercy in every situation. Help me to be willing to trust You in all things. I pray in Jesus' name, Amen.

∽ DAY 23 ∽

Privacy

I grew up in a big family. I had two parents who were not only committed to each other but also their five kids. There was really no such thing as privacy. My parents always knew where we were, what we were doing or who we were with. I had to share a bedroom with a sibling, and don't even get me started on sharing a bathroom! There's no privacy or personal space at all! Believe it or not, I used to hide in a neighbor's doghouse just to get away from people. Inside this space I could read a book in solitude without noise or interruption.

Despite the challenges, it was a blessing to be around so many people who loved me. These types of relationships helped me learn how to connect and get along well with others. The lack of privacy was a little annoying, but that's part of belonging to a big tribe that cared for me and had my back.

Day 23: Privacy

❦ My Journey

Being a young woman isn't easy. Some of us had no idea what we were in for at our first gyno exam. We didn't know how embarrassing it would be to put our legs up in stirrups for a pap and pelvic exam or to let a doctor poke around the most private parts of our womanhood. Frankly, it wasn't until I became pregnant with my son that I became more comfortable with people invading my personal space and privacy. Since the doctors and nurses were professionals, I was sure mine wasn't the only birthing canal they had seen, so I did what I needed to do to bring my two babies into the world.

However, when it comes to being poked and prodded because of breast cancer, it somehow feels more intrusive and the ending is not something beautiful. The continuous disrobing and examination of your boobs by one doctor after another is super uncomfortable. Mammograms squeeze you so hard it feels like you were run over by a car tire. The biopsy can hurt like crazy when they stick that long needle into your chest to snip a couple of samples for testing. Emotionally, it can feel just as intrusive. At every appointment, you're asked a million questions about every personal detail of your life, medical history, and family history— multiple times by multiple doctors. Obviously, these things are very important, but it feels like an FBI interrogation, digging for dirt and trying to find probable cause. When cancer is officially diagnosed, the real lack of privacy begins. Poking, prodding, cutting, stitching, and picture taking are all to be expected. Cancer is indeed a formidable foe. The more information the doctors can get about your history, your family, and the cancer itself, the better the chances of beating this beast. It's just the way cancer works, and we try to get used to it... although we never really do.

✺ Devotional

You have searched me, Lord, and you know me.
You know when I sit and when I rise;
you perceive my thoughts from afar.
You discern my going out and my lying down;
you are familiar with all my ways.

Day 23: Privacy

Before a word is on my tongue you, Lord, know it completely.

You hem me in behind and before, and you lay your hand upon me.

Such knowledge is too wonderful for me, too lofty for me to attain.

Where can I go from your Spirit? Where can I flee from your presence?

If I go up to the heavens, you are there; if I make my bed in the depths, you are there.

If I rise on the wings of the dawn, if I settle on the far side of the sea, even there your hand will guide me,

your right hand will hold me fast.

If I say, "Surely the darkness will hide me and the light become night around me," even the darkness will not be dark to you; the night will shine like the day, for darkness is as light to you.

For you created my inmost being;

you knit me together in my mother's womb.

I praise you because I am fearfully and wonderfully made; your works are wonderful, I know that full well.

Somewhere Between

My frame was not hidden from you when I was made in the secret place, when I was woven together in the depths of the earth.

Your eyes saw my unformed body; all the days ordained for me were written in your book before one of them came to be.

How precious to me are your thoughts, oh God! How vast is the sum of them!

Were I to count them, they would outnumber the grains of sand when I awake, I am still with you. — Psalm 139:1-18

It's comforting to know that the Lord knows everything about us. He knows the good, bad, and ugly and still calls us His own. We never have to worry about being too much or not enough. He meets us in a secret place where there is no need to be private or afraid. We are known and loved in whatever state we present ourselves.

Day 23: Privacy

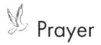 **Prayer**

Father, I am so grateful that there is nothing about me that You don't already know or haven't already seen. When I feel overwhelmed by the intrusiveness necessary for treating this disease, I am comforted in the knowledge that You are with me every step of the way. I thank You for Your constant thoughts and Your perfect solutions in all that lies ahead. I pray in Jesus' name, Amen.

DAY 24

Marked by the Spirit

Being a marked woman has never had good connotations. We read about it in *The Scarlet Letter* as Hester Prynne was marked with an A on her chest defining her as an adulteress. Even as recently as in World War II, millions were put into concentration camps and tattooed with numbers to identify them as Jews. Historically, being marked has been a terrible thing, something degrading to the human spirit-not something easily erased in one's mind or body.

My Journey

We met with a radiologist to do a simulation for my upcoming treatments. I was told my plan would include thirty treatments — six weeks, five days a week. I didn't know what to expect as I went into the simulation. *How is this going to work? Even the word radiation sounds like something out of Chernobyl! I'm not*

Day 24: Marked by the Spirit

sure I'm ready for this. I had no idea how intense and detailed the protocol would be. But I guess that's why they do the simulation!

They made a mold of my chest area by laying a hot, plastic mesh over it. This would be used to hold my body in the exact same place every time I would have a treatment, a safety measure to help avoid accidentally radiating my lungs or heart. The doctor used a permanent red marker all over my chest and underarm to mark the areas for radiation. They measured each red mark carefully and put semi-permanent stickers over the marks to make sure they would line up perfectly with the mesh mold.

Here I was, lying on my back with marks all over my body. More were on the way, as there was still more to be added to the mesh and body stickers. *I know this marking and simulation is necessary to prevent any microscopic cells from spreading, but I still feel like a piece of meat, like part of a dehumanizing science experiment.* Now, every time I look in the mirror at my disfigured chest, I see these red marks and stickers that bring attention to the areas that still contain cells with cancer. I try not to think about the six weeks of treatment I have in front of me or feel the humiliation. I would be lying to say I'm not scared.

☀ Devotional

When you believed, you were marked in him with a seal, the promised Holy Spirit, who is a deposit guaranteeing our inheritance until the redemption of those who are God's possession- to the praise of his glory. — Ephesians 1:13-14

Being marked by the Holy Spirit is a totally different experience. Ever since I became a believer, I have felt marked with the favor of God. It sounds strange, I know, but knowing Jesus has been like having a divine tattoo placed on my heart. Immediately after accepting Christ as my Savior, I felt the Holy Spirit's presence in my life. I never doubted that Jesus was there for me and I belonged to Him. The mark of the Holy Spirit was invisible to the human eye but visible in the ways that He changed me.

Day 24: Marked by the Spirit

But Zion said, "The Lord has forsaken me, the Lord has forgotten me. Can a mother forget the baby at her breast and have no compassion on the child she has borne? Though she may forget, I will not forget you! See, I have engraved you on the palms of my hands" — Isaiah 49:14-16

Instead of seeing our physical marks, we need to remember that we are forever marked in Him by the Holy Spirit. We are loved with an everlasting love, and our names are engraved on the One who bore the nail marks in His hands and feet for our healing. We must remind ourselves that we are sealed and surrounded by the promised Holy Spirit, who is with us and is a deposit guaranteeing our inheritance until our redemption. We are God's priceless possession — to the praise of His glory, and no disfiguring or markings can possibly matter more than that.

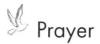 **Prayer**

Father, what a privilege it is for me to belong to You, the One and Only, true God of the universe! I cherish what You have done for me and the price You paid to claim me as Your own. Thank You for putting Your seal on me and help me boldly proclaim that I am Yours! I pray in Jesus' name, Amen.

DAY 25

No Shame

"Shame on you!" That was something many of us heard regularly as we were growing up. Parents in previous generations were very concerned about how their children appeared to others in the community. A child's language or behavior was a reflection on the parents and their parenting style. If a child misbehaved, people would always blame and shame the parents.

With five rambunctious children, it's no wonder my parents were so strict!

My Journey

During one of my deep conversations with my best-friend-and-counselor Becky, I confessed feeling a deep sense of shame connected with this cancer. I couldn't shake the thought that somehow, in some way, I must be responsible for this illness. I hated all the ways it had impacted everything in my life. I didn't want to feel this shame and I wanted to blame something else for this mess. So whose fault was it? I knew my parents weren't at fault because the genetic testing said I didn't have any genetic mutations. It couldn't be God's fault because He's been nothing but faithful and generous to me even when I was far from Him. Blaming Satan would be easy because he's the epitome of everything evil, but what if it was actually me who contributed to cancer forming? I wondered if I could've prevented this whole fiasco if I had changed my eating, exercise routine, or reduced my stress levels earlier in life. Wasn't I the most likely cause of this cancer?

At some level we feel ashamed about who we are. We know that we fall short of who God created us to be. Does that mean we're culpable for our cancer? Maybe, maybe not — who knows? How is it that some who live terrible lifestyles never get cancer, while others like innocent children get it before they even start to walk? There's no way to answer that question. This

Day 25: No Shame

whole line of questioning misses the point: it's not about shame. It's about the Savior.

☀ Devotional

In biblical times, a physical birth defect or an illness would also bring shame. It was a sign of sinfulness.

The opening lines in John's gospel story give us a better perspective of sickness and suffering:

As he went along, he saw a man blind from birth. His disciples asked him, "Rabbi, who sinned, this man or his parents, that he was born blind?" "Neither this man nor his parents sinned," said Jesus, "but this happened so that the works of God might be displayed in him." —John 9:1-3

Jesus focuses not on the cause of the problem but on its purpose. He says the man's blindness was "so the works of God might be displayed in him." If we cling to the shame of cancer and the hardship it has caused rather than focusing on its larger purpose, we will miss the lesson Jesus is trying to teach us. The purpose is to display the works of God in us. That work includes the healing of our physical bodies, but also the spiritual work needed to restore us. This work entails growing in a more intimate relationship with the Father and developing more Christ-like attitudes and behaviors during times of pain or adversity. It means growing our faith and ability to testify of His power to heal, deliver, and save those who believe.

All this is to show who He is — not to showcase the illness we have. It is for the distinct purpose of drawing attention to God, so others will see and believe. This was Jesus' purpose and it's the same for us today.

But we have this treasure in jars of clay to show that this all-surpassing power is from God and not from us. We are hard pressed on every side, but not crushed; perplexed, but not in despair; persecuted, but not abandoned; struck down, but not destroyed. We always carry around in our body the death of Jesus, so that the life of Jesus may also be revealed in our body. For we who are alive are always being given over to death for Jesus' sake, so that his life may also be revealed in our mortal

Day 25: No Shame

body. So then, death is at work in us, but life is at work in you.
— II Corinthians 4:7-12

In the end, having shame about cancer defeats God's intended purpose, and can give a foothold to the enemy. Satan wants us to remain in our shame, to make us feel broken and worthless. Or he wants us to blame God and create distance in our relationship with Him. God, on the other hand, wants to use it to bring glory to His name and display His mighty works in us. Shake off the shame today and declare aloud this truth inspired by Romans 5:

I will boast in the hope of the glory of God. Not only that, but I will glory in my sufferings, because I know that suffering produces perseverance; perseverance, character; and character, hope. And hope will not put me to shame, because God's love has been poured out into my heart through the Holy Spirit, who has been given to me.

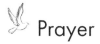 **Prayer**

Father, I come to You in my brokenness, shame, and guilt about cancer and all the dysfunction it creates in my life. I don't want to hold onto any shame because I know this is not from You and does not give You the glory due to You. I confess that I have made this event all about me rather than about giving You an opportunity to show Yourself mighty in my illness. Help me to relinquish my self-loathing and believe You will use every aspect of this to bring glory to Your name. I pray in Jesus' name, Amen.

DAY 26

Just Breathe

When faced with a frightening situation, our heart races, blood pressure rises, and our breathing becomes irregular. It's our body's fight or flight response which happens automatically and takes the situation seriously. In normal, everyday life, fear should not be our default setting. We were designed to rest in the Lord, living in peace with Him and those around us. We were never meant to be in a perpetual state of high alert. That is bondage.

My Journey

The first six days of radiation passed with no noticeable issues, short of being tired from the three-hour drive back and forth every day. To me, it is worth the time and sacrifice to keep going to the University of Michigan for treatment. When I check into the hospital each day, they give me a sticker. I put that sticker on the calendar to mark off how many treatments I've done. It helps me look forward to the last day. 30 days, 30 stickers. My radiology team is great. I call them my "Cancer Killers." Every time I come into the radiation room I say, "Good morning, everybody. How are my Cancer Killers doing today?" They laugh and smile, reminding me just how grateful I am to have them.

It's hard to describe the radiation experience because of the unique feelings associated with it. But it goes something like this:

First, the plastic mesh is taped to my chest. A snorkel-like rubber mouth piece is placed in my mouth and a nose plug is put on my nose to make sure no air escapes from my nostrils. A machine is hooked into the snorkel-like tube to monitor my breathing patterns. A pair of video glasses are placed over my eyes so I can see my breathing pattern on a screen. Finally, I am rolled into an MRI-like tube and they start the radiation. The technicians tell me to hold my breath in the designated yellow area for varying amounts of time, up to 20 seconds while they radiate my marked areas. It takes roughly 15 minutes from start

Day 26: Just Breathe

to finish, which isn't very long, but treatments are required five days per week to be effective. Breathing through a snorkel-like device and having to be completely still takes a lot of concentration. If it is done improperly, the radiation can burn your heart, lungs, or organs. If I had to think about it every day as I went into the tube, I would be terrified. Despite these risks, I get to do it every morning.

I say that I "get to" do this because I am one of the lucky ones. There are many women that don't have the right insurance or access to the information about this treatment option. Even though this is not an easy or painless process, I'll take it all day long and twice on Sunday over chemotherapy! I thank God for medical technology and medical professionals who go the extra mile to make me as comfortable as possible in a potentially dangerous situation.

✸ Devotional

Fear can be healthy in some situations. If we are afraid for a good reason, fear can protect us from doing or saying things that could cause us great harm. However, when fear is unfounded it can paralyze us, cause us harm and be very unhealthy. That kind of fear is never from God. It's a tool of the enemy to make us feel weak and powerless, unable to face our fear.

For God hath not given us the spirit of fear; but of power, and of love, and of a sound mind. — II Timothy 1:7

There is no fear in love. But perfect love drives out fear. — I John 4:18

God is the very definition of perfect love, and as the originator of a pure and holy love, He longs to be in relationship with us. We never have to be afraid because God is always with us. He is our personal "Cancer Killer" and often uses the loving hands of medical professionals to do His work. For every

Day 26: Just Breathe

terrifying procedure that makes us afraid to breathe, we can rest assured that the same God who is ever present in times of trouble will rescue us and breathe His comfort into our spirits. When we call on His name, He's only a breath away.

Prayer

Father, I am the blessed one because I know You and am called Your child. I am allowed the privilege of Your care and the care of those You work through. Thank You, Lord, for my doctors, caregivers, friends, and family who love me and see that I get what I need. Help me to turn to You when I am afraid and know that You love me with an everlasting love and will not abandon me when I call on Your name. Help me to have courage and faith over fear. I rely on You for this strength and thank You for it. I pray all this in Jesus' name, Amen.

DAY 27

Give Thanks

Thanksgiving is the one day set aside and completely focused on recognizing gratitude and blessings in our life. In 2020, I would guess that most people have more complaints than thanks. Even outside of 2020, there have been times this would accurately describe me on Thanksgiving. Nevertheless, for the most part, even amidst the chaos that has been 2020, Dave and I had a lot of little (and big!) things to be grateful for.

My Journey

In January 2020, before the pandemic and my cancer diagnosis, Dave and I took a vacation and drove around southern Florida to visit with friends and family. We ended the trip with a cruise. Austin, Dave's son, passed his PTA licensing test and found his first job as a physical therapy assistant — one

Day 27: Give Thanks

more reason to be very proud of him! During the lockdown, I was able to study for and pass my real estate licensing exam, meaning that Dave and I can work together. Dave's appraisal business had seen new success because of the housing boom and low interest rates, an unexpected highlight of the pandemic.

My son, Ryan, and his wife, Holly, welcomed a sweet baby girl, Lucy, to the family. Many of our family members were exposed and tested positive for COVID, but no one has been severely impacted. My parents live in a care facility and are considered high risk, but we are very grateful for FaceTime and technology to keep in touch every week and help them not feel so isolated.

When I received my diagnosis, it rocked any kind of stability we had established while going through the other turbulent events in 2020. But, God has never left us! Prayers and support have poured in and we have seen miracles in the storm. I had excellent doctors, a successful surgery, and an answer to prayer with a low oncotype score. Not needing chemotherapy was a blessing in itself! We were so grateful for all the help that my daughter, Lacey, and her husband, Dave, offered with weekly grocery shops, cleaning, and setting up a meal train. We were grateful for selfless friends who offered up meals, talks on the phone, homes for me to stay during treatment and hundreds of acts of service to help us cope during such a stressful time. Even though the circumstances of 2020 have been less than stellar, we were so very lucky to reflect on the year from a lens of gratitude.

☀ Devotional

Give thanks in all things, for this is the will of God for you in Christ Jesus. — I Thessalonians 5:18

We experience God's faithfulness and goodness toward us in so many ways. We shouldn't wait until Thanksgiving to give voice to our gratitude, but seek out ways to recognize blessings every day, week, or month. We know we have been held in the palm of our awesome God's hand, the One who knows what we need before we even say a word. He provides

Day 27: Give Thanks

everything for us as we offer Him our unspoken prayers. We are humbled by His care for us and His work through the many hands of those around us. Thanks be to God who is so worthy to be praised — today and every day! What are you thankful for today?

Prayer

Father, I could never praise You enough for who You are and what You've done for me. I praise You in the small and big ways You have blessed me. If You never did another thing to show Your care for me, I have received more than I deserve or could ever repay. Forgive me, Lord, for the times I overlook Your mercy and grace. Forgive me when I become arrogant and think I deserve more than I have received. Help me to be grateful in all things, even if it isn't always what I want or think I should have. Help me to always believe that You are good and faithful. I pray in Jesus' name, Amen.

∽ DAY 28 ∾

Waiting for the Promise

Growing up, Christmas at my home was always a big deal. It centered around Advent and the birth of Jesus, but it was one of the few times that us kids could look forward to getting a gift. With such a big family, gifts were not frequent or a priority. I remember my sister finding one of the hidden presents, opening it up to peek at its contents, and then resealing the paper as if she had not seen it at all. She just couldn't wait for Christmas to come, and I know how she felt. I can't wait for Christmas to come and for radiation to be over!

🎗 My Journey

It's December 16th and Christmas is only a few days away. Since mid-November, I have been doing radiation every day. I'm starting to see the light at the end of the tunnel and the final week, week six, is around the corner. I feel like Rudolph with

Day 28: Waiting for the Promise

his glowing red nose, only I'm Lindy, the Red Chested Lady with the weird, glowing red boob!

No, my glowing headlight doesn't save Christmas or do anything heroic, but I do get to be finished after seven more treatments. Hopefully, my red radiation rash will go away quickly, there won't be any complications, and my skin will begin to heal. That would be the best Christmas gift I could ask for! During this time, Dave and I were very careful about where we went and who we saw because of the pandemic. We stayed in and decorated our house with our old decorations and shopped for gifts online. Something I didn't want to get for Christmas? COVID! My radiation care plan wouldn't play nicely if I had to quarantine, and I simply could not risk getting sick and stopping treatment. This time of waiting was all leading up to Christmas, where we could finally gather with loved ones and live some type of "normal" life.

Our season of waiting also coincides with Advent — a time that Christians observe as a season of preparation for the birth of Jesus. Most of 2020 has felt dark and ominous. During this time of waiting, we looked to Jesus as a bright light in our dark world. The light of our Savior cannot be dimmed by cancer, COVID, economic insecurity, loss of loved ones, or any other tragedy. As we waited for treatments to be completed, we were ever mindful of the One who spoke light into the darkness from the beginning. In Him is life and that life is a light to all people. Together we say, "O come, O come Emmanuel!

Devotional

For to us a child is born, to us a son is given, and the government will be on his shoulders. And he will be called Wonderful Counselor, Mighty God, Everlasting Father, Prince of Peace. — Isaiah 9:6

The Word became flesh and made his dwelling among us. We have seen his glory; the glory of the One and Only, who came from the Father, full of grace and truth. — John 1:14

The Advent season reminds us where our hope, joy, peace, and salvation come from. Jesus is our Wonderful Counselor,

Day 28: Waiting for the Promise

the One who sees us and our individual circumstances and guides us through every day. This gives us abundant hope. He is a Mighty God who formed us and is able to heal us. This fills us with love for Him. He is our Everlasting Father, from now to eternity, no matter what. Jesus is our Prince of Peace, the One who came to bring peace and reconciliation to all people. This allows us to rest in Him even when our world seems crazy. I am so grateful that He is our Emmanuel, "God with us." He has come as a light in the darkness and the darkness has not overcome Him.

Prayer

Jesus, You are the One I long for. You are the One whose birth is the answer to everything I need. Thank You for being my light in the darkness that cannot be overcome. Thank You that COVID, cancer, despair, chaos, or any work of the enemy must flee because of Your great name. It's in the name above every other name that I pray, Amen.

DAY 29

Ring the Bell

As a child, I distinctly remember how we were called for dinner. One of our tribe of five would go outside and ring a cowbell throughout the neighborhood to alert the rest of us that dinner was ready. We lived in Iowa during a time when children would freely roam miles from home without much worry. Wherever we were, we would stop what we were doing and come running home to eat. This bell announced something important was happening and you'd better pay attention, or you would miss it — and go to bed hungry!

My Journey

This past week, on my last day of radiation treatment, I got to ring the bell. Six weeks of traveling, thirty days of dressing and undressing to get this treatment, and now I can relax! I'm sure it was far less intense and invasive than chemotherapy would

Day 29: Ring the Bell

have been, but it was not without cost. There will still be months of healing for my blackened and peeling underarm and breast. There will be lots of lotion and sleepless nights trying to find a comfortable spot where it doesn't hurt to roll over. There will be a period of adjustment before I can continue with my reconstruction efforts, but ringing that bell was a significant milestone. It's the announcement of an important event. I have done everything humanly possible to rid my body of this cancer and I declared that I am healed, in the mighty name of Jesus!

While undergoing treatment, it is natural to keep a stiff upper lip and just push through to do whatever you have to do. There's no time for complaining or drama — just do it and get it over with. After radiation was complete, Dave and I had our own kind of emotional breakdown. It felt like the intense hormone crash after having a baby. You go through 40 weeks of pregnancy, manage pain during labor and delivery, and when it's all over you cry tears of joy and relief as you hold the blessed reward of your suffering. Dave and I didn't get a little one out of this, but we cried tears of joy for this part to be over, and tears of relief because I made it through without infection, expander failure, or COVID. We did everything known to man to finish well, and we have! There will be no looking back and second guessing ourselves. We are so grateful for the staff at the Cancer Center and my Cancer Killers in the radiation oncology department. We are also very grateful for family and friends and the meals, house cleanings, cards, visits, gifts, and prayers from so many. It's the difficult times that have shown us who our tribe really is!

On Christmas Eve, I rang the bell to signify victory over cancer and announce that we are never going back...NOT EVER! The Christmas song, "Ring the Bell" was one I learned as a child. Its words announce the birth of our Savior, Jesus Christ. I have received healing because of a baby lying in a manger. We all have the opportunity of new and eternal life because of this gift. So, ring the bell, sing the song, and celebrate this milestone with us. More importantly, ring the bell for Jesus! If you miss that, you'll miss more than dinner.

Day 29: Ring the Bell

✳ Devotional

Ring the Bell! Ring the Bell!
Let the whole world know
Christ was born in Bethlehem, many years ago.
Born to die that man might live.
Came to earth new life to give
Born of Mary, born so low, many years ago.
God the Father gave His son, gave His own beloved One
To this wicked, sinful earth to bring mankind His love, new birth
Ring the Bell! Ring the Bell!
Let the whole world Know
Christ the Savior lives today as He did so long ago!

Prayer

Jesus, we celebrate Your birth in this Christmas season, while also acknowledging it was to provide a way for our salvation through Your death. Without You, I would still be lost in my *sinfulness. I know that my healing only comes because of Your grace and mercy upon me. Thank You, Father, for allowing me to celebrate victories, but help me never to forget to give You the glory for what You have done through Christ Your Son. Amen.*

> Are you enjoying SOMEWHERE BETWEEN?
>
> Be sure to write a review on Amazon!

DAY 30

Seize the Day

Carpe Diem! This saying was popularized by Robin Williams in an old movie called, *Dead Poets Society*. It was a brilliant film about seizing the day and living life to the fullest with no regret. Very few people I know leave this earth, completely satisfied with how they lived or without any regrets. I too, will likely have couple of regrets before I die but seizing the day will not be one of them!

My Journey

After I rang the bell to celebrate completing my radiation treatments, Dave and I decided it was time to take a vacation. Since it was winter, the only places I wanted to consider were warm ones! *Do we want to fly or drive, stay in one place the whole time, or travel around and see more? There are so many choices!* We finally have a get-out-of jail-free card after being *trapped in the house for so long. Yes, COVID is still a factor and wearing a mask won't be fun, but so what? I am alive and done with cancer!* We just wanted to have some fun!

We decided to take a road trip from Michigan to Florida, making lots of stops along the way. We planned a packed agenda: Kentucky to see Churchill Downs, North Carolina to stay at The Cove in the Billy Graham Center, South Carolina for a pit stop in Charleston, and a walk down cobblestone streets in Savannah, Georgia. We experienced a variety of warm Florida venues, hanging out with friends and family along the way.

Ten days into the trip, we were exhausted and wishing for naps by the time the clock struck noon. We had seized enough days. We weren't sure if it was the sudden surge of activity after being locked down for so long or the after-effects of radiation which caused the fatigue, but this time cancer had not robbed us of the enjoyment of life. We were grateful for this time together and we smiled as we headed home and thanked Him for His vacation provision.

Day 30: Seize the Day

✺ Devotional

The LORD is my shepherd, I lack nothing.
He makes me lie down in green pastures, he leads me beside quiet waters, He refreshes my soul.
He guides me along the right paths for his name's sake.
Even though I walk through the darkest valley, I will fear no evil, for you are with me; your rod and your staff, they comfort me.
You prepare a table before me in the presence of my enemies.
You anoint my head with oil; my cup overflows.
Surely your goodness and love will follow me all the days of my life,
and I will dwell in the house of the LORD forever. — Psalm 23:1-6

We all need times of restoration. God wants to give us times of enjoyment in the midst of our troubles. This is especially true for those of us who are always in the valley of the shadow of death. We take His blessings gratefully and thank Him for these times of refreshing! We never know when or if cancer will throw us another curve ball, so we do our best to receive His grace, mercy, and favor.

We should never feel guilty about the money or time it takes away from our family and friends to have a vacation. Instead, we must allow the overflow of God's goodness to saturate us fully so that we can face the next chapter of our journey. We live here on earth only once, so if we enjoy some precious relaxation and revelry, let's do it with all our might as unto the Lord.

Prayer

Father, I praise You because every good and perfect gift comes from You. The rest You provide for my weary soul is truly a gift. I am keenly aware that life is but a vapor, and we are only on the earth for a short time. Help me, Lord, to enjoy everything that I experience. Help me to embrace You and Your creation,

Day 30: Seize the Day

to appreciate Your restoration and ever-present goodness. I bless You and thank You for it all in Jesus' name, Amen.

DAY 31

Walkie Talkie

There was a time when cell phones were non-existent, and people actually had to go next door to talk to their neighbors or get in the car and drive across town to find out how someone was doing. When the drive was too far, there were handwritten letters to communicate important information or well wishes. We have lost some of the intentionality and intimacy of face-to-face encounters and I'm not sure it's been a good thing.

My Journey

Dave and I have developed a habit of taking long walks together nearly every day. Initially, we started doing this because we were trying to lose some weight. We began with a short route around our neighborhood, but eventually we were walking a good distance at a decent clip. Whether it is

Day 31: Walkie Talkie

raining, snowing, windy, or blazing hot, we are committed to our "walkie-talkie" together. It gives us time to decompress from the day and talk about whatever.

At this point in life, the primary focus of my conversations is on two things: work or cancer. We are in the real estate business, so as we walk around the neighborhood, I'm usually talking about our clients, new homes on the market, homes I'd like to get on the market, or homes that are not yet ready for the market. Pair that with talk about cancer studies, treatments, and upcoming appointments — our walkie-talkies can quickly turn into doubty-pouties. As you can probably imagine, this hasn't always been enjoyable for Dave. He can get weary listening to me rattle on with such a limited agenda when we could be talking about more positive things like our blessings and the beautiful nature around us.

❋ Devotional

Luke 24 shares the story of two men on the Road to Emmaus. These men were walking back to their hometown talking about all the events surrounding the crucifixion of Jesus which had happened just days earlier. They were discussing the reports they had heard about His resurrection and doubting their authenticity. Then, Jesus appeared and started walking with them, discussing the prophecies surrounding these events. They didn't recognize Him until sometime later in the evening in a very poignant moment.

When he was at the table with them, he took bread, gave thanks, broke it and began to give it to them. Then their eyes were opened and they recognized him, and he disappeared from their sight. They asked each other, "Were not our hearts burning within us while he talked with us on the road and opened the Scriptures to us?
They got up and returned at once to Jerusalem. There they found the Eleven and those with them, assembled together and saying, "It is true! The Lord has risen and has appeared to

Day 31: Walkie Talkie

Simon." Then the two told what had happened on the way, and how Jesus was recognized by them when he broke the bread.
— Luke 24: 30-35

The road to recovery on this cancer journey can consume all our thoughts, feelings and energy. It's a bit sad how oblivious we can be to the people and events happening around us when cancer becomes our focus. We become myopic in our perspective. Just like these men on the Road to Emmaus, when we allow ourselves to be consumed by doubt, negativity, or worry, we fail to recognize the truth, beauty, and relationships that matter most. We miss the broader picture of life.

Find some time today to intentionally look for new ways of appreciating the beauty and people around you. Try something you never thought you'd do. It might be painting, bird watching, blogging, or going somewhere new with friends. See if it doesn't open up a new avenue for growth in your personal or spiritual life.

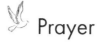 **Prayer**

Father, I acknowledge that often I fail to notice all the beauty that surrounds me. I fall into the trap of seeing with limited vision and focusing on things that don't point to You or Your goodness. I often miss out on other things You intend for me to enjoy. Help me, Lord, to recognize the blessings You so freely give and the opportunities to see where You are at work in the world. Open my eyes, Lord. Give me new vision and a heart that burns within me for Your truth. In Jesus' name I pray, Amen.

DAY 32

Scars

Every mom or dad has probably watched one or more of their children running full speed down the street, only to trip and fall. They plummet to the ground, scraping their faces, hands, elbows, or knees. This traumatic event is inevitably followed by a stream of tears, all-encompassing hugs, and multiple kisses of boo-boos. Sometimes these wipeouts cause minor scrapes, while other times there will be scars.

No one gets out of this life without scars. Everybody has them. Some are so pronounced you can't help noticing them. They tell a story of wounding, pain, and recovery that could leave the victim permanently and publicly disfigured. You don't want to stare, but your eyes are drawn to the area of trauma. You wonder what happened and perhaps even cringe at the thought of what it must be like to live with this indelible record of offense.

Other scars are so small that they are hardly noticeable. The event which caused the scarring appears to be so minor that it doesn't impede the wearer at all. Nevertheless, it's still a scar. Still others are hidden beneath the surface and never see the light of day. These are the internal scars that plague people daily, wrought by emotional trauma that may or may not have been intentional. They are an ugly disfigurement to the soul brought to life as external scars, but a smile or well-developed denial system can make them invisible to the average person.

ribbon My Journey

Cancer leaves scars in all sorts of places. The mastectomy left a scar twelve inches long on my chest. Every day, I see the incision doing its best to heal. Its dark red, jagged edges remind me the tumor is gone, but so is part of what makes me look like a normal female. I am lopsided and there's no getting around that.

Day 32: Scars

Dave has never been afraid to see my scars and has never cared if I had or would ever have a breast. He loves me no matter what, and just wants the cancer to be gone. Not every woman is blessed enough to have a Dave in their life. I suppose I will get used to the incision line and the small expander underneath. Eventually the expander will be full and the scar should fade, but for now all I can see is the rawness of it all, the drain tube coming out of the side of my chest and the ugliness of what cancer has done to my body. Even though Dave and I can see it, thank God no one else can.

✤ Devotional

He was despised and rejected by mankind, a man of suffering, and familiar with pain.
Like one from whom people hide their faces he was despised, and we held him in low esteem.
Surely he took up our pain and bore our suffering, yet we considered him punished by God, stricken by him, and afflicted.

But he was pierced for our transgressions, he was crushed for our iniquities;
the punishment that brought us peace was on him, and by his wounds we are healed. — Isaiah 53:3-5

Jesus endured the torturous beating, the nails that pierced His hands and feet, and the sharp sword that pierced His side. He was publicly humiliated and maimed for us. If He had recovered from this torture, He surely would have had scars. But these injuries killed Him. His mortal body couldn't survive this type of punishment, yet when He received His heavenly body, the reminders of His suffering were still there. These scars were to His glory, not His shame.

Now Thomas ... one of the Twelve, was not with the disciples when Jesus came. So the other disciples told him, "We have seen the Lord!" But he said to them, "Unless I see the nail marks in his hands and put my finger where the nails were, and put my hand into his side, I will not believe."
A week later his disciples were in the house again, and Thomas was with them. Though the doors were locked, Jesus came and

Day 32: Scars

stood among them and said, "Peace be with you!" Then he said to Thomas, "Put your finger here; see my hands. Reach out your hand and put it into my side. Stop doubting and believe."
Thomas said to him, "My Lord and my God!"
Then Jesus told him, "Because you have seen me, you have believed; blessed are those who have not seen and yet have believed." — John 20:24-29

We all bear the scars of our suffering. Whether they're physical, emotional, or spiritual scars, these should not be our shame but a reminder of God's sacrifice for our ultimate healing. We can be grateful for our scars because they were purchased at a high cost — by His stripes we are healed.

🕊 Prayer

Father, I come to You with deep sadness because I see the scars that remind me of the brokenness I feel. There's a sense of loss and shame for not being as whole as I want to be. As I grieve, the loss reminds me, Holy Spirit, of how Jesus was battered, beaten and scarred for me. He lost all of His dignity to heal my brokenness both inside and out. Help me reframe how I view my own scars. Help me to see them as representations of necessary losses leading to healing through His sacrifice. Rather than identifying with the world's understanding of what is feminine, help me find identity and wholeness in Christ. I pray In Jesus' name, Amen.

∽ DAY 33 ∽

Intimacy

Everyone loves a good love story. It usually begins with a spark between two people that leads to a special connection. This may be an emotional, spiritual, or physical experience but unless these things are developed within a committed relationship, they will never lead to true intimacy or a real love story. Intimacy is intentional and usually developed over a long period of time. It's not a short-term venture.

⚑ My Journey

Dave and I were both in our late 50s when we met online. We were a perfect match from the start. We openly shared our likes, dislikes, hopes, dreams, faith, and everything we thought would be important to talk about in developing our relationship. It was in some ways more like an interview than a dating thing because neither of us had a desire to date. We were both looking for a mate. When we eventually met for the first time, the physical spark was there and the rest...well, you know. We were married a year and a half later and couldn't be happier.

We had no idea that within another year we would be navigating the challenges of cancer. No one told us this would seriously mess with our sex life, and my desire would switch from "Let's go!" to "Heck no!" The change was stunning. The fatigue of treatment and the effects of the hormone suppressors immediately threw my body into super menopause mode. The side effects were extreme and produced bone pain, dryness, and depression like I'd never known.

There were only two options. Take the hormone suppressor with all the side effects and have a 15% recurrence rate in the first three years, or refuse and have no side effects, a better sex life, and the risk of a 30% recurrence rate. The choice was clear! All the same, the change in sexual libido presents a serious learning curve for any spouse, especially when you're newly married.

Day 33: Intimacy

When you compound all of that with looking in the mirror and seeing the ugliness of losing a breast, the scar that reminds you of what you've been through, and the fear that your husband will be repulsed by the sight of you, it's no wonder no one wants to tell you the truth about how hard it's going to be.

☀ Devotional

In the beginning when God created Adam and Eve, there was nothing but perfect unity and intimacy in their relationship with each other and the Father. After the Fall, however, everything changed. Genesis 3:24 tells us that Adam and Eve hid from God because they were afraid, naked, and ashamed. The tactics of the enemy had successfully broken the intimacy they had with each other and with God. Satan's strategy hasn't changed. He is still using the same game plan today.

When the effects of cancer make us afraid or ashamed of our nakedness in front of our spouses, we fall victim to that trap. Intimacy is broken. Sexual intimacy is a representation of the sacred spiritual union of two becoming one, and we cannot allow cancer or any of its effects to tarnish our self-image or destroy our spiritual and emotional connections with our spouses and God. We must refuse to allow the enemy to get a foothold in our marriages. Instead, we bring our fear, shame, and broken bodies before God and ask Him to redeem all of it for His namesake.

Thankfully, Dave and I have rebounded. Statistically, we're probably still in the top tier of sexually active folks our age, but all jokes aside, I'm super grateful that we're still all about it. (Sorry, to our adult children. We know you didn't want to read that!) We're old but we're not ready to give up the ghost just yet.

Dave and I have found new ways of compensating for the difference. We talk about the changes and how we can accommodate each other. We take advantage of longer warm up times and have learned to embrace the new normal, which isn't really that different now that we've made the adjustments. I thank God for an amazing husband who sees me for me, and

Day 33: Intimacy

who has built a strong foundation of emotional and spiritual intimacy with me that will overcome anything cancer has thrown at us. This is what makes a true love story and brings abundant blessing.

Prayer

Father, You are the creator of all things good, and I thank You for that. You want me to have a deeply intimate connection physically, emotionally, and spiritually with You, as well as my spouse. Help me, Lord, not to be afraid of how my body looks after cancer. You see me for who I am, so help me make fear and shame disappear in the light of Your love. Please help my spouse make these big adjustments to enjoy deeper intimacy in spite of our struggles, and to be patient with me in the process. I pray for Your grace and mercy in Jesus' name, Amen.

∽ DAY 34 ∾

Connection

A few of you may be old enough to remember the Jetsons, the cartoon family of the future who went places in flying vehicles, had robots do their housework, and could see people as they talked through their computers. This was a dream in the 1960s. Today, it is our reality. Working from home through video calls and even telemedicine has become common practice. While all this is convenient and fantastic at some level, it also has a downside. People have lost tangible opportunities to connect with their families and communities.

✿ My Journey

While undergoing radiation treatment, Dave and I were intent on doing whatever was necessary to avoid contracting COVID. Attending church, seeing family and friends, and unnecessary activities were all put on hold to decrease my risk

Day 34: Connection

of infection. We were concerned that if either of us got sick, it would stop me from completing all the treatments. We were perfectly content to be in our little bubble at home and only leaving the house to go to the hospital and back. It made us feel safe.

Now that my treatments are over, there is a glaring awareness of the social disconnect created by the pandemic. We had traded an active, vibrant life for safety and missed a lot. Connections are hard to maintain in general, even more so virtually, and equally as hard to resume once they've been neglected. God made us to be relational and function in community. It was of great importance to Him and should be to us as well.

☀ Devotional

From the beginning, God said in Genesis 2:18-22, *"It is not good for man to be alone,"* so He made Eve as a companion for Adam. No one was meant to go it alone!

In the book of Acts, communicating and gathering in faith communities was quite difficult. Persecution was severe and yet, these early disciples of Jesus found ways around their circumstances. They did not allow fear to deter them.

Every day they continued to meet together in the temple courts. They broke bread in their homes and ate together with glad and sincere hearts, praising God and enjoying the favor of all the people. And the Lord added to their number daily those who were being saved. — Acts 2:46-47

During the pandemic, fear caused people to withdraw from fellowship instead of pressing into it. They felt depressed and isolated. Children couldn't go to school, massive mental health issues emerged, and suicide rates skyrocketed. Marriages dissolved at an alarming rate. Gun violence and crime plagued the nation, all due to the fear of sickness and physical connection. I believe this was the enemy's most evil attack— to keep us away from each other, to make people feel fearful and vulnerable.

Day 34: Connection

In order to reestablish our relationships, we needed to find ways of reconnecting. Dave and I decided we can be careful and still interact in a small community. We started going out, attending church, and meeting with people in intentionally wise ways. It was scary at first but now we are more comfortable, taking calculated risks, and getting our lives back. We refused to let COVID determine how we connect with others.

How have your life and relationships changed because of cancer? What steps can you start taking to reestablish community again?

Prayer

Father, I confess that I have been fearful and worried about my illness. I've been trying to protect myself and others from illness, so much so I have neglected my relationships with those You have put in my life. I want to be wise and careful, so help me, Lord, not to fear the tactics of the enemy. Help me to reconnect with You and others who follow hard after You so that I can maintain our emotional and spiritual strength in the face of many trials. I command fear, depression, anxiety, and every demonic stronghold which raises itself up to a place of authority in my life to bow to the name of Jesus and to leave me right now. I give first place to You, Lord, and I ask You to restore my social and emotional connections so I, like the people in Acts, can have a heart full of praise and favor with all the people. I pray this in Jesus' name, Amen.

DAY 35

Leftovers

You can find them in most people's refrigerators- leftovers from the night before. They make for a quick, convenient dinner or lunch, when I remember to eat them! While some are too delicious to waste, others are stashed in the back of the fridge and when they are finally discovered, they look more like your kid's slimy green science experiment than any dinner I've ever cooked. Most of the time I don't mind leftovers – they make my lunch prep so much easier. When I forget they exist, I wish I could throw them out without having that signature Dutch guilt. When it comes to what my friend, Sharon calls, "cancer leftovers," there are more science experiment kinds than lovely second day delights.

🎗 My Journey

It has been three months since my final radiation treatment. To be honest, my recovery progress was a little disappointing. One of my "leftovers" included taking a daily hormone suppressor. My oncologist says cancer feeds on female hormones, so depending on which hormones it prefers (estrogen, progesterone, or Her2), a hormone suppressor can help starve any residual cancer cells, making it difficult for them to grow again.

Since my recurrence rate without the hormone suppressors is so high, taking them for the next 5 to 10 years is a no brainer. While the decision was clear based on my doctor's recommendations, the side effects are less than ideal. The suppressors throw your body into super menopause mode. *Really, doc? As if the typical hot flashes, night sweats, lowered libido and mood swings weren't enough! My bones and joints hurt, too. Add the Omegas, calcium supplements and other vitamins, and I feel like a walking pharmacy!*

Day 35: Leftovers

We thought that we were on track to establish some type of new normal and get started on reconstruction, but we were mistaken. These are not the carefree, sunny days that we dreamed of, but they also aren't completely gloomy or without positivity. It's part of post-cancer recovery and life. We aren't always going to get what we want or feel like the world is on our side (spoiler: it's not!) but we can control our attitude. The enemy wants to speak words of anxiety, discouragement, distraction, and doubt in our ears. It's easy to see the road to recovery as unending and question whether the radiation was enough to kill every bit of microscopic cancer. Who knows if I'll have to face this beast again someday! Only God knows and He is for us even in the leftovers.

❋ Devotional

Praise God we don't have to wait for a physical reunion with the Lord to have peace! He is present here and now.

Peace I leave with you, my peace I give to you. Not as the world gives do I give to you. Let not your hearts be troubled, neither let them be afraid." – John 14:27

Before Jesus left the earth, He also declared to His disciples in Matthew 28:20, *"I am with you always…even until the end of the age."*

He didn't leave us to face our disappointments alone but sent the Comforter in His place to be with us, speak peace into our souls and guide us into all truth. We need the presence of the Holy Spirit every single day of our life. Thankfully, we can meet with Jesus anytime we want for worship and prayer. We never walk alone but are always in the hollow of His hand.

 Prayer

Father, You and You alone know every emotional and mental process I go through with each new day. You care about every one of these things and how they affect my life. But where I see

Day 35: Leftovers

obstacles, You see avenues. Help me to bring all expectations to You and filter them through not only the realities of what can be seen on the surface, but what You say about them. Continue to help me see Your goodness, faithfulness, and sovereignty in the difficulties as You speak peace. I pray this in Jesus' name, Amen.

DAY 36

Copays

Growing up Dutch, I was taught to be very frugal. We never wasted anything and saving money was top priority. We lived debt free and didn't need to keep up with the Jones'. We didn't have a lot of toys, but we had everything we needed and a few fun things we wanted. It was a stress-free way to live. Life is a lot different than that today.

My Journey

Cancer makes a mess of your finances and dealing with insurance issues can be as frustrating as dealing with cancer itself. When you have a modest household income, getting good insurance without a high deductible is next to impossible. If you can manage to do that, then there's this annoying thing called a copay. I'd like to meet the genius who dreamed that up! It's hard enough dealing with a life-threatening illness but

Day 36: Copays

harder still not to feel angry and a little resentful that cancer has taken thousands of dollars from our families, and we still have thousands more to pay!

Dave and I made a commitment early on in our marriage to tithe the first tenth of our income to our church. I only say this because it's our privilege to give back to God's Kingdom a small portion of what we've received. Truthfully, it's all God's money anyway so we are blessed to keep ninety percent to take care of our needs and a few wants. The frustration comes when the amount we owe in copays and deductibles is more than what we give as our tithe. We want to give so much more to Kingdom work and faith-based causes but are stuck handing over our hard-earned dollars to hospitals and treatment facilities. It seems so unfair!

❋ Devotional

When I think back on my spiritual journey, my questions about finances used to be very different. *What if I tithe on my income and don't have enough money for my daily needs? Why should I give away money that I can use to save for my future or buy things I needed?*

Now my thinking has changed and I'm sad that we can't give more! What caused this paradigm shift?

"Bring the whole tithe into the storehouse, that there may be food in my house. Test me in this," says the Lord Almighty, "and see if I will not throw open the floodgates of heaven and pour out so much blessing that there will not be room enough to store it. I will prevent pests from devouring your crops, and the vines in your fields will not drop their fruit before it is ripe," says the Lord Almighty. "Then all the nations will call you blessed, for yours will be a delightful land," says the Lord Almighty. – Malachi 3:10-12

Over the years, we tested the Lord as we gave our tithe and discovered His faithfulness in bringing us through every difficulty. While He has not rebuked the cancer devourer or kept other hardships away from us as we had hoped, He has provided ways for us to stay afloat and has blessed us in

Day 36: Copays

innumerable ways. He knows we need money to run our home well and pay for treatment, and we have no doubt He will provide. If we continue to trust God for His provision, we will continue to see that we can trust Him in every area of our lives. We are convinced we can never out-give God.

The Lord knows the intentions of our hearts. How much money we give into Kingdom focused initiatives isn't the issue. Giving joyfully and sacrificially is what's important. Even the jobs and finances we have been given are gifts from His hand. It's all about being faithful in our giving, even if it's much less than we would want to give.

Prayer

Father, You are incredibly good to me and generous in all You do. I thank you for the medical professionals that You have brought into my life to help me recover from cancer. Bless them today. I also thank You for every dollar that You provide for me to get the treatment needed and pay for copays and deductibles. God, I know You own everything and are perfectly capable of giving me exceedingly, abundantly more than I could ever ask for or imagine. I love You and appreciate my job, my family, and everyone that has sown seed into my recovery. I know this, too, is from Your hand. Help me, Lord, to trust You with my finances, to give joyfully, graciously, and sacrificially into Your Kingdom despite our circumstances. I trust You to do even greater things for me than You have already done. I pray in Jesus' name, Amen.

DAY 37

The Exchange

One of the first things you need to do when entering another country is to visit a currency exchange. There, you'll discover an exchange rate, which determines how much money you get for your money. You can lose or gain value in the exchange depending on the current rates and fees. The end goal is to get what you want without paying too high a price. That's how it feels with an implant exchange.

My Journey

Ten months had passed, and we were nearing the time to exchange the expander in my chest for an implant. However, in that time period, we noticed some unusual changes to my scar that not only had us concerned, but my doctors as well. As my scar widened, I brought it up to my doctor and was told the last five radiation treatments, called a "scar boost," were focused directly on the scar area to prevent any cancer from coming back in this area. These treatments had thinned my skin and the scar was dangerously close to reopening to expose the expander. If this happened, the result would be emergency surgery.

Because of these new developments, I was told I needed to wait a bit longer to do the exchange. We held our breath and prayed for no additional complications. During the waiting, Dave asked if I was sure I wanted to continue with reconstruction. I thought it over and decided that what would be best for me is to finish what I started. I had already spent months in pain and didn't want it to be for nothing. When the day came for the surgery, I couldn't have been more ready. I was happy to exchange the hard, painful plastic expander for a softer, more flexible new breast. The cost of waiting was painful, but I hoped the result would be what I wanted.

Day 37: The Exchange

✸ Devotional

The Lord is in the business of exchanging good things for things that are broken.

He bestows on them a crown of beauty instead of ashes, the oil of joy instead of mourning, and a garment of praise instead of a spirit of despair. – Isaiah 61:3

We can fully expect the Lord to redeem and restore us. He wants to exchange all the rotten things that the enemy has heaped on us with blessing and good things from His hand. We can be confident that our good and loving Father will not make us wait any longer than necessary to give us His best. He will do everything in His time and it will be beautiful in His sight. We are the recipients of an amazing exchange — Jesus' life for ours. God sacrificed His own Son, Jesus, in exchange for our sin, sickness, and redemption. We paid nothing but it cost Him everything. It's a divine exchange that's scandalous. That's the extravagant love of God.

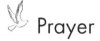 **Prayer**

Father, I give You all the glory for the amazing ways You have blessed me with Your overwhelming grace, love, and favor. You take every negative and turn it into a positive just because You can, and You delight in doing so. I have nothing in and of myself that is of value or can be equal to what I receive from You; but, Father, I give You what I have. I give You my praise, gratitude, and whole heart as I thank You for Your heart toward me. Help me to remember Your sacrifice for me and the blessings I receive because of it. I ask this in Jesus' name, Amen.

DAY 38

Unexpected

Have you ever come around a corner at the exact moment as someone else and you nearly collide? Your first response is to pull back, startled by their presence, apologize, and move on. With cancer, you learn to expect the unexpected. You begin to expect that around every corner, there is the potential for collision.

My Journey

Another day, another wake-up call about the ongoing effects of cancer. I slept peacefully but I woke up to a bed full of liquid and a rupture in the scar of my newly reconstructed breast. It was shocking. I thought, *"What is this?? I am three months out from the last reconstructive surgery and on my way to normal. This can't be good!*" In the weeks following my implant surgery, I experienced a bit of pain and pressure in my chest but dismissed it. Must be part of the process! Now, this could not be ignored.

It's not uncommon for radiated skin to be so damaged that it becomes thin and unable to heal or withstand anything that could cause breakage. The pressure from fluid build up had become too much for the scar to contain so it came out at the point of least resistance. We called the surgeon immediately and went to the University of Michigan to get this checked out. My reconstructive surgeon said an open wound was an invitation for infection. The implant was exposed, so it was recommended that it be removed. She asked if I wanted to try again with a new implant.

After weighing all the factors, it just didn't make sense. *I don't want to go through this over and over with no guarantee that it will be any different later. Burned skin is burned skin. Even without an implant, the process of healing could take a year or two! No, thanks, I'll pass!* I am so disappointed with the result, but I tried my best. Two days from now I will have another surgery and be a one-boob wonder again. *Will this ever be over?*

Day 38: Unexpected

❋ Devotional

In I Samuel 1, we read about the disappointment of a barren woman named Hannah. In biblical times, not being able to bear children was not only disheartening but shameful. We don't know why the Lord had closed her womb, but we know her infertility was part of His plan. Hannah's husband had another wife named Peninnah who had many children and was cruel to Hannah, provoking her to tears because she was infertile. Can you imagine what that would be like? She must have questioned God's plan for her life.

Barrenness was not only a sign of God's disfavor but also a black mark on her womanhood. Hannah cried out to the Lord and promised to dedicate any child she would conceive to the service of the Lord. Then something unexpected happened. It was miraculous. After years of disappointment Hannah bore a son, Samuel, who would serve the Lord as a great priest and prophet in Israel.

Disappointments take time to work through. It's not easy to continue grieving when it seems like one loss after another.

Bring your disappointments to the Lord and tell Him everything in your heart. He won't turn away but will comfort you. God closes doors for a reason and opens new ones in due season. We aren't always going to know why. God is God and, though He doesn't owe us an explanation, He isn't callous or uncaring when we hurt. With cancer, we have to expect the unexpected and hang on to the faithful God who walks with us, comforts us in our pain and shame, and never leaves us empty-handed. He provides what we need when we need it, even when it doesn't happen in our timing.

Prayer

Father, I confess that I don't always understand Your ways, but You tell me in Your word that my thoughts are not Your thoughts and my ways are not Your ways. Your ways are far above my ways. I know this is true. When I am disappointed in what life brings, help me to remember Your sovereignty. Nothing comes to me unless it first goes through Your hands. I belong to You,

Day 38: Unexpected

Lord, and will trust You even in the unexpected. Help me submit to Your will and way. I pray in Jesus' name, Amen.

∽ DAY 39 ∽

Hospital Hoopla

As a kid I watched a tv show called Emergency and was spellbound by the crowd of medical professionals that raced to the scene of trauma. They moved at lightning speed to make sure the injured person had every opportunity to survive and recover. I decided at a young age that I wanted to be the youngest neurosurgeon in the world. As you now know, it didn't turn out that way, but I maintain a great deal of respect for those who practice medicine and make it their life's work. What would we do without them?

🎗 My Journey

I was preparing to have my implant removed, never suspecting the next forty-eight hours would be like Mr. Toad's Wild Ride! I was getting ready for my upcoming surgery to have my implant removed, and just before, I came down with a fever,

Day 39: Hospital Hoopla

chills, and pain in my chest. Dave and I immediately recognized that this was most likely the infection we had hoped to avoid. We immediately drove to the emergency room in Ann Arbor, where Dave was turned away due to COVID precautions. Unhappy, but realizing there was nothing we could do, I went in and Dave waited (not so patiently!) and prayed.

After eight hours of IV antibiotics, blood and fluid cultures, they took me to the operating room and successfully removed the implant. Generally, they would send you home the same day for this procedure, but they couldn't take the risk of sending me home with an unresolved infection, so I was assigned a hospital room. Dave was able to visit before he drove back to Battle Creek to get some sleep.

The next day, the infection was still being cultured and doctors didn't know how long it would take to have the pain and bacteria under control, so the surgeon decided I should stay longer. She planned on prescribing something to treat the infection at home for two weeks, but we experienced some roadblocks due to an allergy. There was one other option or being sent home with an IV antibiotic. For those of you who know me well, you know that being cooped up in my house with an IV antibiotic would be the worst possible scenario. It would have all the makings of a Life Time movie called, *Crazy Town—She Didn't Mean to Murder.* Thank God the second treatment worked!

☀ Devotional

What do we do when everything gets turned upside down and there's no control of the situation we find ourselves in? The most common response is to cling desperately to the small things we can control or throw up our hands and become victims of the process – neither of which are ideal. Perhaps we should listen for a moment to the words of the Psalmist:

God is our refuge and strength,
an ever-present help in trouble.
Therefore we will not fear, though the earth give way
and the mountains fall into the heart of the sea,

Day 39: Hospital Hoopla

though its waters roar and foam
and the mountains quake with their surging.
There is a river whose streams make glad the city of God,
the holy place where the Most High dwells.
God is within her, she will not fall;
God will help her at break of day.
Nations are in uproar, kingdoms fall;
he lifts his voice, the earth melts.
The Lord Almighty is with us;
the God of Jacob is our fortress. – Psalm 46:1-7

Read through a few Psalms today and find one that gives you comfort and encouragement. We don't have to be victims. We are more than conquerors through Christ Jesus.

Prayer

Father, when I find myself in frightening and unpredictable waters, I confess, Lord, that I want to be in control. I want to have a say in what happens to me. I forget that I am incapable of controlling the world around me. But You are more than able. Jesus, help me to remember that You are the creator and sustainer of everything in this world. You are my fortress in times of trouble and, more importantly, You are with me. I ask You to calm my heart and speak peace as I navigate rough waters. I pray this in Jesus' name, Amen.

~ DAY 40 ~

Room for Others

It's been said that strangers are just friends you haven't met yet. I guess it all depends on how willing we are to welcome someone into our space. Some strangers are stranger than others.

✤ My Journey

While I was in the hospital, I had two roommates. The first time I heard Christina's voice, it was from behind a curtain. I couldn't see her face, but I knew she was smiling just by hearing her voice. At first, I didn't know why she was there, but over the course of the night and the following day, I got to hear her story and learn more about who she was as a person.

Although we were from different cities, had different backgrounds and different diagnoses, we were far more alike than different. Turns out we were both believers, had been single parents, were relatively conservative, and even shared the same birthday! She talked about her interest in real estate, and we promised to keep in touch. It was a lovely, divine encounter that I am still grateful for.

Christina was discharged later that day and a new patient arrived. Let's call her Martha, for storytelling purposes. Martha stayed behind her curtain the entire night and next day, never really speaking except to complain. She was demanding of the nurses and her aroma was so pungent that it made me wish for wide open cow pastures.

The reason I don't know Martha's real name is because I never asked. I just didn't care enough to reach out and get to know her. That fact alone made me stop and check my heart. Did I care for Christina more because she was engaging and fun to be with even during an illness and disregard the other woman because she was hard to stomach? *Why didn't I have compassion for her the same way I did for Christina? What if God avoided or was apathetic toward me because I was whiny, demanding, and stinky in my attitudes or physical body?*

Day 40: Room for Others

I sometimes wonder how I would feel if God dismissed me the same way I dismissed her.

The physical space was small in that hospital room, but I hadn't left any emotional or spiritual space for my neighbor. I wondered what kind of opportunities I had missed by failing to see her as a person of worth. Suddenly, I realized I wasn't really a very good neighbor either.

☀ Devotional

In Luke 10:25-37, a teacher of the law is trying to make himself feel good about his own righteousness, and Jesus confronts him with a story. A man was lying on the road after he was beaten and robbed by thieves. The priest and Levite disregarded the dying man and walked on the other side of the road to avoid becoming ceremonially unclean. Then a hated Samaritan, who had no status or obligation to help, had pity on the dying man. He not only took him to a safe place for medical care and help but paid for it as well. This man was merciful and that's what made him the "Good Samaritan."

There are times when we are all apathetic or indifferent toward others. Even when we want others to be kind and empathetic toward our situation, we aren't always the same in return. It's easier for us to excuse our attitudes and behaviors because we get tired of dealing with our own stuff. Maybe we've pulled the "cancer card" and tuned out when we should've been more engaged and compassionate with everyone around us.

Jesus said that when we care for the least of those around us, it's like caring for Him. Perhaps we need to periodically check ourselves to see how we are doing. Do we try to justify our own goodness, or do we need to check our own levels of compassion?

 Prayer

Father, it is so easy to engage with those who are like me but dismiss those with whom I don't seem to have anything in common. Help me to see people the way You do, Lord, to see

Day 40: Room for Others

their value as individuals You love and created. Help me not to avoid those that are difficult to engage with. Help me get to know them and their stories. Give me humility in listening, grace in responding, and love for everyone You put in my path. Help me share Your love with them, too! I pray this in Jesus' name, Amen.

༄ DAY 41 ༄

Stay in Step

Follow the Leader is an old game with very basic rules: there is a leader who decides every step and several followers to trail behind. The leader is in complete control of the game. They may move quickly or slowly. Their movements may be jerky or awkward, but it doesn't matter. The object of the game is to do whatever the leader says to do. The followers' job is to stay in step with the leader.

🎗 My Journey

There's always a step-by-step process in fighting cancer. First are the tests, then the diagnosis followed by the plan of treatment, which has more steps and follow-ups for the steps to make sure you're on the right path. The truth is, doctors can only give you the next step when they see how your body responds to the last. No one has a crystal ball and they are just

Day 41: Stay in Step

making their best educated guess based on best practices and experience.

When I had my first surgery, we had no idea they would later find microscopic cancer in my lymph nodes or would be unable to get clear margins as they removed the tumor. If we had known my skin would be so burnt it would damage the inside of my chest cavity and I would not be able to heal well, we would never have opted for immediate reconstruction. We would have taken a different direction and waited until after radiation to consider it. If we'd known how good prosthetics were, we might have decided on no reconstruction at all. At the time, we took what we thought was the next right step with the information available to us.

Sometimes I wonder, *who or what is leading us in this journey? Is it the cancer and doctors, or fear of COVID, or some other threatening circumstance?* If I'm honest, I must confess it hasn't always felt like the Lord. Occasionally, I allow my thoughts to go into the "what ifs." I listen carefully to everything the doctors recommend but don't always spend enough time listening to what the Spirit is whispering in my ear. There are times when I act out of self-protection, my own timeframe, or selfish desires rather than allowing the Lord to go before me and be my rear guard. It's not easy to be a follower. It takes a lot of trust and you're never quite sure if you've made the right choices.

☀ Devotional

The Psalms and Proverbs are Old Testament books of poetry and wisdom. Many of the Psalms begin as laments and contain deep questions from the writers' souls, but usually end with encouraging words about the Lord's faithfulness. Proverbs contains 31 chapters of wise instruction, one for every day of the month. This makes it easy to read one chapter a day and glean all kinds of wisdom for every situation we may face. Cancer or not, we all need wisdom.

Trust in the Lord with all your heart and lean not on your own understanding; in all your ways submit to him, and he will make your paths straight. – Proverbs 3:5-6

Trust in the Lord and do good;

Day 41: Stay in Step

dwell in the land and enjoy safe pasture.
Take delight in the Lord,
and he will give you the desires of your heart.
Commit your way to the Lord;
trust in him and he will do this:
He will make your righteous reward shine like the dawn,
your vindication like the noonday sun. - Psalm 37:3-6

The Lord makes firm the steps
of the one who delights in him;
though he may stumble, he will not fall,
for the Lord upholds him with his hand.
I was young and now I am old,
yet I have never seen the righteous forsaken
or their children begging bread.
They are always generous and lend freely;
their children will be a blessing. – Psalm 37:23-26

If we want to know how to follow the leader and keep in step with the Lord, we only need to turn to God's Word for direction.

We readily have it at our disposal and if we take the scriptures seriously, they will speak truth into our lives.

 ## Prayer

Father, in the midst of my questions, doubts, fear, or regrets, help me to trust You. It is difficult to hear Your voice when there are so many voices trying to influence my decision making. I don't want to lean on my own understanding but want You to lead me in everything I do. Help me, Lord, to delight in You and trust You to lead me in the right way. Help me not to be dual-minded, but to follow You as You lead me in paths of healing. You have everything mapped out for good and will bring it forth as I follow hard after You. Thank You for Your guidance and wisdom. Keep me in step with You as You lead the way. I pray these things in Jesus' name, Amen.

∽ DAY 42 ∾

Gratitude

My mom taught me social graces like saying please and thank you. I'm sure there were times when I said thank you simply because it was required of me and not because my heart was truly grateful. It was the polite thing to do regardless of my attitude, but gratitude is an essential part of a happy and prosperous life in any circumstance.

❦ My Journey

Every time I sit down to write an entry, I get very emotional. Today I'm a grateful, emotional mess. If the last sixteen months have taught me anything, it's to cherish every day, every experience, and memory; to be present and grateful for what I have, not what I want.

Somewhere Between

Through the years I have wanted a lot of things, mostly things that are self-serving and make my life more comfortable or easy. We think an easy life is always a blessed one, but it just isn't so. An easy life is preferable, but it can make us complacent, self-centered, and entitled. It can deceive us into believing we are the center of the universe and deserve to be favored. It can make us self-reliant rather than reliant on God.

Challenges, however, bring us to a place of humility. They put us in a position of uncomfortable insufficiency, not knowing how we are going to press through the hardship by depending more on our own resources. For me, it's what has built my dependence on God, on others around me and reminds me that I am not self-sufficient, but exactly like everyone else. We are not alone in the battle. Struggles can make us grateful or bitter. At some point in life, we all choose the lens we will see life through and the attitude we will have. The good news is this: Even if we choose to be bitter for a season, it's not permanent. At any time, we can change our minds and choose an attitude of gratitude instead.

Day 42: Gratitude

In truth, there are days when I get worn down and weary dealing with cancer and the hardships it brings. I look toward heaven and ask: *Lord, could you give Dave and I a break? A win, just for once?* Within minutes, however, I am convicted of my ungrateful attitude. What if just being alive and surviving three surgeries, a massive infection, and a global pandemic at the same time is a win? What if having a wonderful husband, great doctors, an awesome family and supportive friends is God's favor — His win for me? This shift in thinking changed my perspective, showing just how much I have to be grateful for!

On the other hand, what if suffering, recurrence or the threat of death is God's ultimate plan? Should I be less grateful?

✺ Devotional

Real faith and gratitude say, "Whatever you think is best, Lord." Is it easy? No. These words may be some of the hardest. It means that we surrender our will and let God have His way in our lives, no matter what the outcome may be. Gratitude is a posture of grateful submission to the One who owns our mind, body and soul. In life or death, easy or hard, we are called to gratitude.

Read Psalm 138 aloud. Make it your offering of gratitude to the Lord.

I will praise you, Lord, with all my heart;
　before the "gods" I will sing your praise.
I will bow down toward your holy temple
　and will praise your name
　for your unfailing love and your faithfulness,
for you have so exalted your solemn decree
　that it surpasses your fame.
When I called, you answered me;
　you greatly emboldened me. – Psalm 138:1-3

Though I walk in the midst of trouble,
　you preserve my life.
You stretch out your hand against the anger of my foes;
　with your right hand you save me.
The Lord will vindicate me;
　your love, Lord, endures forever – Psalm 138:7-8

Day 42: Gratitude

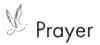 Prayer

Father, I come to You today without any agenda at all. I don't come to ask for Your grace, protection, provision, or anything else that I need. I am fully aware that You have already provided everything I need as I have needed it. I come to simply and humbly say thank You for who You are. I seek You and not what You are able to give me. You and You alone are more than enough. I am grateful to know and be known by You and for the privilege of being called by Your name. Help me to remember to be grateful in every situation, knowing everything that comes my way passes through Your loving hands before it ever gets to me. Keep me humble and open to whatever You have in store for me. I pray this in Jesus' name, Amen.

∽ DAY 43 ∾

COVID and Caregiving

Ring Around the Rosies is a silly childhood game we used to play. We had no idea this song was describing the 14th century Bubonic Plague which caused the deaths of thirty plus million people and wiped-out half of Europe's population. As kids, we would form a circle, hold hands, and joyfully sing these words as we rotated around in a circle. "Ring around the Rosies, pocketful of posies, ashes, ashes, we all fall down." The song would end with us all on the ground, laughing hysterically. But there was nothing funny about it when it was a reality.

⚘ My Journey

The pandemic took everyone by surprise being the first pandemic the world had seen since the 1918 Spanish flu. In December 2019, before anyone knew what COVID was,

Day 43: COVID and Caregiving

Dave and I were both seriously sick and coughing uncontrollably for nearly six weeks. In January 2020, the facts started to come out about this virus and the panic began. There was a lot of anger, fear, finger pointing, and mandating; but none of it halted the virus.

In November 2021, nearly two years later, Dave and I both caught the virus again, but a different variant. We had every symptom listed! Everyone was worried about me because I had just completed my third surgery and had a compromised immune system, but Dave had it worse than me. It started with us both taking care of each other, but with each passing day, Dave got more and more sick. He had a terrible cough, low oxygen levels, and a debilitating fatigue that made him sleep upwards of twenty hours each day. It lasted nearly a month! My mind was screaming, *What if I can't take care of him? Please God, don't let him die!* I was terrified of losing him. When you are already sick and need to care for someone who is much sicker than you, it changes your whole perspective on caregiving.

Those who care for others often end up getting sick themselves. They focus on the one who is ill and meeting their needs, instead of taking care of themselves. It's a common problem. I only got a small glimpse of what Dave had been experiencing as he took care of me for the past year and a half. I'm sure he was worn out and tired, worried about what the next day would bring, and feeling helpless. I'm sure he too, was terrified of me dying and being left alone to deal with all the grief and aftermath. Caregiving isn't for the faint of heart and I have such a new appreciation and respect for Dave and all the other caregivers of the world.

☀ Devotional

Bear one another's burdens and so fulfill the law of Christ.
– Galatians 2:6

Cast your cares on the Lord and he will sustain you; he will never let the righteous be shaken." – Psalm 55:22

These verses tell us we must care for others and be cared for at the same time. Caregivers need to be able to take a step back, have some down time, and delegate the responsibility of

Day 43: COVID and Caregiving

caregiving to a select group of others they can trust to do what needs to be done. It is imperative for their mental, physical, and spiritual health. No one can be everything for someone else. That is God's job. We are all merely human beings who are ourselves in need of God's care. Allowing time for rest, taking restorative time with the Lord or doing things you enjoy is not selfish. It is necessary self-care in order to be better equipped to care for others. When a caregiver can cast their cares on the Lord, they will find more strength, energy, and peace than they thought possible. Another one of those blessings in God's economy!

Encourage your caregivers to take some time for themselves. Whatever that looks like for them, it is an important part of caring for others. It doesn't have to be something big, although it can be, but needs to be something that gives them time-out from their day to day reality. Pray for them as they pray for you!

Prayer

Father, Thank You for always caring for me. At times I lack the energy and resources to care for myself, let alone care for others who are in need. I need Your strength to push through and Your peace for my weary soul. Enable me by Your Spirit to lean into and receive care from Your hand as I care for myself and others. I pray this in Jesus' name, Amen.

DAY 44

Build Up

If at first you don't succeed, try, try again. It's an adage that my parents and their friends taught their children, encouraging them to persevere in the face of hardship or defeat. Children have a natural tendency to be resilient, but with every new failure, disappointment, or discouragement, negative attitudes can build up. If they don't learn to persevere, walls of defeat can become permanent barriers to their success. Dysfunctional patterns from childhood can be crippling in adulthood. Not all of us have learned to be resilient, but cancer gives us the opportunity to build up these skills.

My Journey

After a severe bout with COVID, I had a check-up, and some new complications were discovered. A large pocket of fluid called a seroma was found in my chest cavity. I felt a little bit of pressure in my chest, but again, thought it was part of the healing process. The incision was healing nicely, but the cavity was full and squishy instead of concave like it was supposed to be. I could push on one side of my incision and see a wave of fluid pushing to the other side of it.

The formation of a seroma was surprising. The surgeon couldn't tell whether it had formed because of COVID inflammation or my previous infection, but we had to address it. The solution was to put a long needle in my chest, drain all the fluid, apply deep compression and hope the tissue would heal. *Ouch!* I was told to wear a compression vest 24/7 to see if this could help. After four weeks of check-ups, four weeks of continuous fluid build ups and four weeks of fluid aspirations, our hopes for a normal recovery are dashed. I'm trying, but I am tired. Tired of trying and trying again.

Day 44: Build Up

✸ Devotional

Carrying the heavy burden of cancer and recovery is not what anyone is intended to do. The enemy wants to pile one trouble on top of another to make us weary and despondent. He wants to build walls of resentment, hopelessness, and defeat in our souls so that we will stop fighting, believing for healing, and proclaiming victory in Jesus' name.

Come to me, all you who are weary and burdened, and I will give you rest. Take my yoke upon you and learn from me, for I am gentle and humble in heart, and you will find rest for your souls. For my yoke is easy and my burden is light. – Matthew 11:28-30

Jesus knows our disappointments and invites us to partner with Him to lighten our load. When we become yoked in relationship with Jesus and learn how to work with the Holy Spirit, our burdens become lighter. We begin to understand His gentle hand in our lives and experience His humble heart for us. It is in Him that we find our rest and in His strength that we are enabled to push through and try, try again. Whenever you feel a setback, remember that the Lord is building up resilience in you. He is helping you to get back up again and partner with Him in your next step to victory.

Prayer

Father, it is so easy for me to see everything that seems wrong in my life, so I forget to focus on what is right. Disappointments, delays, and unexpected detours should not impact me so much; but they do. Help me, Lord, to reject the negative, and embrace my relationship with You. Your heart's desire is for me to be healed, but also for me to be satisfied in You and You alone. I ask You to break down any walls of resentment or disappointment that would separate me from You and Your blessing. Build me up in Your most Holy Spirit, so I might run this race with stamina and courage. I pray all this in Jesus' name, Amen.

∽ DAY 45 ∽

New Year Old Truths

Ringing in the new year is a time-honored tradition in every nation and people group on the planet. Devouring dumplings, racing to eat the first grape of the year, or kissing the person next to you at midnight – each of these joyful, cultural traditions has their place in the celebration. New Year's Eve gives closure to the old year and ushers in the potential for a new beginning and the hope of something better.

🎗 My Journey

We had a couple of crazy years in 2020 and 2021, so in 2022, no one is looking for a trilogy of trauma. Everyone is looking for something new, something better. They are looking for a new relationship, a new job, a better routine or something they think will improve their lives. They want to get back to "normal" and find a rhythm again so things can be easier, less stressful and more convenient. But not me!

Sure, those things are great to think about, and sometimes it seems like those things will make everything right with the world. The truth is, nothing but an old truth will make things right with the world. It's one I have held onto for more than twenty-five years: Jesus is the only One who can make a difference. He's the only one who can revive a weary soul, give peace, provide the things we need, heal our physical and mental brokenness, and save our sin-sick souls.

Every time I look to other things to satisfy my needs, I am always disappointed and frustrated. I walk away empty-handed and inevitably return to the true source of life and eternal life. There's nothing else. Believe me, I've tried pretty much everything known to man, and all of it pales in comparison to the magnificence of the Lord our God.

Soon, I will undergo my fourth and, hopefully, final surgery. I'm told this next step is necessary for a full recovery from the effects

Day 45: New Year, Old Truths

of reconstruction. I'd like to believe my life will be easier and the doctors will be able to stop the continuous fluid that keeps building up in my chest cavity. I'd like to think there is some magical pill or potion I could take to make this seemingly never-ending garbage go away, but it always comes back to this old truth. My faith and trust is in the God of the universe, the One who made every cell in my body, who has written every day of my life in the book of life, before it ever came to be.

☀ Devotional

Everything eventually comes back to these words from Psalm 46:10. The scriptures below were adapted by Anne Graham Lotz and expanded by me. They're thoughts I have adopted to begin this new year.

Be Still and Know That I Am God – See Psalm 46:10

BE STILL

Be quiet

Switch off my Phone ~Listen

Somewhere Between

Stop commenting, arguing, questioning or complaining

AND KNOW

Be confident, stop doubting, be sure, have faith

That I AM GOD

The Almighty, In Control

Loving, Compassionate

KING of HOPE

Faithful Father that Restores Me

Provides and Protects Me

Now and Forever.

That's where we'll find healing and hope in 2022.

Prayer

Father, I proclaim this to be a year of health, hope, and quiet confidence in Your goodness. I ask You to help me stop all the unnecessary activities, thoughts, and verbalizations that keep me from hearing or seeing You for who You are. I dedicate myself to drawing closer to You as You draw closer to me. Help

Day 45: New Year, Old Truths

me, Lord, to have increased faith, hope, and love for You and all those around me. Do a new thing in me today. I pray in Jesus' name, Amen.

DAY 46

Hope in the Crushing

When it's January in Michigan, there are snow piles as far as the eye can see. Every time I get the mail and a breath of fresh air, I can hear the crunching of the snow beneath my feet. It's the hearty kind of snow that's great for making snowballs and snow forts. When you crush it together in your hands, you know it's going to stick together and become like a hard, impenetrable rock that isn't easily broken. This is what we've been hoping for with my seroma pocket.

My Journey

It's a little unreal to me that three weeks have passed since my last surgery. The time has gone both very slowly and very quickly — if that makes sense. My surgeon told us this time they really put the hurt on me to make sure the fluid stopped accumulating. She scraped out the chest cavity and all the scar

Day 46: Hope in the Crushing

tissue again, then cauterized the skin around it and sutured the seroma pocket down to the pectoral muscle. She topped it off with a nice chest tube to drain out any fluid that might try to accumulate again – the works! When I woke up in recovery, the pain was like excruciating. The first week was a blur but thankfully, the pain subsided during week two as healing started to take place.

I wore a compression vest 24/7, taking it off only to shower. It's like a pretty tube top I pack with gauze to compress the chest area, which is once again concave. This compression is supposed to help the tissue heal properly, but wearing it means that most of the time I feel like I'm being squeezed to the core! I know this uncomfortable bit of crushing must be working because a few days ago the fluid accumulation in the drain bulb was so small they removed my chest tube! Hopefully, this will be the end of surgeries and the beginning of true and lasting recovery.

✳ Devotional

Before Jesus was arrested, He went with His disciples to the Garden of Gethsemane to pray. The word "Gethsemane" means olive press, which is a solemn foreshadowing of what was to come in terms of Jesus' arrest, trial, crucifixion, and ultimate resurrection.

In biblical times, the olives were crushed, then pressed for different and distinct purposes. The olives first had to be crushed by a large stone to begin the process of obtaining the oil. The crushed olives were then put in the olive press and a heavy stone was placed on top of the basket of olives. The pressure squeezed out the oil which ran down into collection vats.

The first time the olives were pressed and gathered, the oil was used in the lamps of the temple to give light (Exodus 27:20). It was also used for anointing oil (Exodus 30:24; James 5:14) and for meal offerings (Leviticus 2:4-10). The second time the olives were pressed, the extracted oil was used as healing medicine (Isaiah 1:6; Luke 10:34). The third press rendered

Day 46: Hope in the Crushing

oil suitable for making soap and cleaning mixtures (Job 9:30; Jeremiah 2:22; Malachi 3:2).

He was wounded for our transgressions, he was bruised for our iniquities: the chastisement of our peace was upon him; and with his stripes we are healed. – Isaiah 53:5

We are hard pressed on every side, but not crushed; perplexed, but not in despair; persecuted, but not abandoned; struck down, but not destroyed. We always carry around in our body the death of Jesus, so that the life of Jesus may also be revealed in our body. – II Corinthians 4:8-10

This crushing is not pleasant – it's painful! Jesus was crushed too, but it was for us and our healing. We count it a privilege to be identified with the One who took the crushing for us.

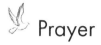 **Prayer**

Father, I come to You with a deep sense of gratitude for all the ways You have sacrificed for me. You took my sin and sickness, guilt and shame, redeeming it by Your blood. You did this for no other reason than Your great love for me. There's nothing in me that is worthy of Your sacrifice and nothing I can do to repay You for what You've done. So I fall on my knees before You and give You the only thing I have: my heart. Thank You for offering Yourself to me and accepting me as Your child. Help me to walk worthy of the high calling You've given those who bear Your name. I pray in Jesus' name, Amen.

～ DAY 47 ～

Using Wisdom

I haven't always been very good at making choices. I'm either impulsive and jump into things way too quickly or have a bad case of analysis-paralysis. My recklessness has led to many regrets, while my over analyzing has caused me to fear mistakes and kept me stuck in unhealthy places. There are so many decisions to make when it comes to this cancer journey. It's not like picking a flavor of ice cream to enjoy. Many choices are literally life-threatening and one bad choice can kill you. Using wisdom is a challenge.

☬ My Journey

It had been months since Dave and I stepped foot, physically, into a church. We were watching online every week, but it's not the same. We were being careful about exposing ourselves to the virus again, especially with a new variant on the rise. We know that even people who are triple vaccinated and those like us with natural immunity are still getting sick. We want nothing to do with that, especially since thousands of people attend our church for weekend services. *We have to be wise — but what is wisdom?*

Of course, we want to be there with our church family, serving on the Prayer Team, taking our grandkids to service when they spend the night with us, but there's so much to consider. *Should we go in late, wear a mask the entire service, avoid talking with people and jet out of there as soon as the last amen is said? Or should we throw caution to the wind, gather with our families, friends, and church community and trust that somehow everything will be alright?* We needed wisdom!

☀ Devotional

While Proverbs is known as the Old Testament Book of Wisdom, James is often referred to as the New Testament Book of Wisdom.

Day 47: Using Wisdom

If any of you lacks wisdom, you should ask God, who gives generously to all without finding fault, and it will be given to you. But when you ask, you must believe and not doubt, because the one who doubts is like a wave of the sea, blown and tossed by the wind. That person should not expect to receive anything from the Lord. Such a person is double-minded and unstable in all they do. – James 1:5-8

Wisdom comes from God and He wants to help us make good decisions about our health, treatment, and life in general. We try to figure it out for ourselves, but our wisdom falls miserably short of the wisdom God wants to generously give us. The key is our willingness to ask. When was the last time you intentionally took some time to pray, fast, read, and get Godly counsel?

It takes humility to go to Jesus and admit we don't have all the answers. Often, we're stuck in our own unproductive thoughts about what's right and wrong. It takes an open heart and ears to listen for His response, instead of rushing in headlong and taking our chances with the outcome. If we will do what it takes to hear His voice, we will have peace in the decision-making process. If not, we will be unstable in all our ways.

 Prayer

Father, I come humbly to You today, seeking wisdom in choices. You can speak to me and guide me in the right path for my situation if I will turn to You and ask. I don't have Your eyes to see where I should go or what I should do, but I trust You to help me make good decisions. You know my heart is to be in community with others, to love and serve You so please help me, Lord, not to be afraid. Help me listen for Your direction, and believe without doubting, so my life will be stable as I make choices in line with Your will. I pray all this in Jesus' name, Amen.

༄ DAY 48 ༄

Checking In

Every Sunday, we get on a video call with my parents. Between cancer and the pandemic, it's been nearly a year since we've traveled to Iowa for a visit. They are in a senior care facility, so for a long time they were in lockdown and couldn't have any visitors. These weekly calls have been one of my greatest joys amidst the sadness of not being able to see them in person. I take comfort in the technology that has allowed us to see each other, but it's not the same as being there. Still, it's our weekly time to share news, support each other and stay accountable.

Accountability is a word not everyone likes. It can feel like an obligation, but realistically it's more like a blessing. Having doctors, family, and friends to keep me accountable is a rare thing. When left to my own devices, my mind can be as dangerous as a NASCAR race track with thoughts flying around at unprecedented speeds. My emotions can spin out of control and there's always the chance to crash and burn. Having a pit crew of people is exactly what I need. They keep me aware of my progress and prepare me for the dips, bumps, and curves along the way. They keep me on track for a successful finish. Check-ins are a necessary part of the process, but they only work if they're done with transparency and consistency.

☒ My Journey

Several weeks after my final surgery, my surgeon examined my chest, poked around a bit and declared the surgery a success. *Hallelujah!* I had been diligent about being still, wearing my compression vest, and not doing anything that would jeopardize the process – basically, following all the doctors' orders- which is progress for me! It had taken a long time and a team of people to help me get to this place, but the hard work and resilience finally paid off.

Day 48: Checking In

The check-ins along the way were the accountability I needed to help me make the necessary adjustments and finally achieve success. And for that I'm very thankful!

☀ Devotional

Two are better than one; because they have a good reward for their labor. For if they fall, the one will lift up his fellow: but woe to him that is alone when he falleth; for he hath not another to help him up. Again, if two lie together, then they have heat: but how can one be warm alone? And if one prevails against him, two shall withstand him; and a threefold cord is not quickly broken. – Ecclesiastes 4:9-12

Accountability is not only good when you're dealing with cancer – it's necessary in all areas of our lives. It's easy for us to think we can handle things ourselves and slide down the slippery slope of self-sufficiency, but that is the beginning of the end. If we reject accountability, our own denial systems, pride, or the whispers and schemes of the enemy, it can derail us before we know it.

Somewhere Between

Accountability is modeled for us as we look at the Trinity. In John 5:30, Jesus makes Himself accountable to the will of the Father:

I can of mine own self do nothing: as I hear, I judge: and my judgment is just; because I seek not mine own will, but the will of the Father which hath sent me. – John 5:30

Jesus says this about the Holy Spirit as well:
But when he, the Spirit of truth, comes, he will guide you into all the truth. He will not speak on his own; he will speak only what he hears, and he will tell you what is yet to come. He will glorify me because it is from me that he will receive what he will make known to you. All that belongs to the Father is mine. That is why I said the Spirit will receive from me what he will make known to you. – John 16:13-15

Accountability and humble submission is a must. There is no room for pride. If we make the Lord our team leader and are accountable to Him first, we cannot fail. How are you doing as a team player? If you're having difficulty checking in and being accountable to the Lord or your pit crew, take some time today

Day 48: Checking In

to delve into that and discover where the problem is coming from. When you find the issue, take it to the Lord and ask Him to help you realign. It is the fastest way to success.

Prayer

Father, it is with gratitude and humility that I give all of myself to You. I am fully aware that my own thoughts and resources are not enough to keep me on the right track. I need You to be my everything. I submit my life and will to You and thank You for bringing others to travel with me along the road to recovery, to help keep me on the straight path. Thank You for modeling through the Trinity what it means to be in divine community. Help me be willing to use this model in my own life to draw closer to You and others. I pray this in Jesus' name, Amen.

DAY 49

Prosthetics

I am amazed when a well-known actor takes a role that makes them look nothing like their real self. The makeup and prosthetics they wear literally transform them into someone who is unrecognizable to their fans. This is done in movies for the sake of a specific look or character. When it comes to cancer, prosthetics are there to make us look normal and more like our natural self, not less.

My Journey

After my incision from my first mastectomy surgery in 2020, I decided explore purchasing a prosthetic. Even with an expander in my chest, I was still a bit lopsided and I didn't like the way my clothes were fitting. I also wanted to get one for my swimsuit because that would be even more noticeable. I didn't want to look odd to others and I wanted to feel normal, even if

Day 49: Prosthetics

I knew I wasn't. I looked online and found a place called Beautifully Unique. This shop not only sold prosthetics but a variety of clothes, swimsuits, and accessories for women with breast cancer. I had never heard of a shop like this and was intrigued, so I made an appointment.

The ladies there were wonderful and fitted me for what I needed. I was stunned at how natural the fake boob felt and it even had a nipple! I had no idea how close a prosthetic could be to the real thing or how much better I would feel wearing it. Isn't it strange how we somehow feel less female if we don't have the lady-bits that femininity traditionally requires? Why do we think a pair of boobs complete us? And who do we need to prove our femininity to?

Now in 2022, and I'm starting over again. Since my reconstruction failed and there is no breast tissue left in my concave chest, so I need a new prosthetic or something else to fill in the gaping cavity. I've heard of a few options and might pursue them, but I'm now in a place where I know who I am regardless of whether I have a breast or not. God sees and knows it's still me, so if I don't feel like wearing a prosthetic and people think I look weird, that's okay; I'm over it.

☀ Devotional

As ye have therefore received Christ Jesus the Lord, so walk ye in him: Rooted and built up in him, and established in the faith, as ye have been taught, abounding therein with thanksgiving. Beware lest any man spoil you through philosophy and vain deceit, after the tradition of men, after the rudiments of the world, and not after Christ. For in him dwelleth all the fulness of the Godhead bodily. And ye are complete in him, which is the head of all principality and power. – Colossians 2:6-10

The world tells us we are less than because we have a missing or misshapen breast, but as Christ followers we know that the only One who has the authority to judge who we are is Christ alone! We are not less feminine because we have lost a body part. We can walk in His fullness and be thankful despite our loss.

Day 49: Prosthetics

Our bodies aren't who we are. They are just physical tents we live in until we leave this earth and get our new bodies. I know that ultimately, we will be made new. The only thing that truly matters is being solid in our faith, not swayed by the opinions or philosophies and ideas of the world. We hold only to Jesus and who He says we are in Him: Beloved, Accepted, Redeemed, and Complete in Him!

Prayer

Father, by Your word, You created all things. You have the power to restore any part of my body that has been lost. But when that's not in Your plan, You carefully and lovingly provide a way for me to function as You had intended, and to feel whole. Thank You for modern technology that makes it possible to replace body parts lost through accidents, sickness, or disease. I am blessed by Your care for me and thank You for helping me realize I am much more than my physical body: I am Your precious child and in You I am complete. Thank You

Somewhere Between

for Your grace upon me. Keep me in Your loving care, in Jesus' name, Amen.

~ DAY 50 ~

Sabbath Rest

I learned about Sabbath rest from my parents. Sundays in the DeBoer house were considered a day for doing nothing except going to church in the morning, taking a nap in the afternoon, and going back to church for evening worship. To be honest, I didn't like Sundays much. I thought they were super boring. We were not allowed to do any of our normal weekly activities on Sundays. I couldn't ride my bike, play with my friends or even watch TV, except for maybe a football game. I had a lot of energy and didn't think I needed a rest – but with five active kids I'm sure my parents did!

⚘ My Journey

As I've gotten older — and maybe a little wiser! — I have come to realize that God knew exactly what He was doing when He gave Moses 10 Commandments and included the command to "observe the Sabbath day by keeping it holy." (Deuteronomy 5:12). Sabbath rest is probably the best gift God ever gave people. It was something He Himself modeled for us after the creation was completed. He knew that rest was good for our bodies, minds, and spirits.

In the process of overcoming cancer, I've gained a lot of respect for the value of rest. I used to have a great deal of difficulty taking a stop day, a time of Sabbath rest to be present with the Lord. Now after eighteen months of surgeries, pain, and healing, I'm a whole lot better at embracing the very thing that used to make me lose my mind — being still. I doubt I will ever go back to that hamster wheel of life I was on for so many years. Believe me, you can even be on it while doing ministry and think you're doing great exploits for God while disobeying His command to rest on the Sabbath. It happens to the best of us.

Taking a Sabbath has also given me time to look back on my journals and ponder the work the Lord has done in me. It's something I would never have done unless I was forced to. Today, I thank God for the opportunity to reflect on the ways

Day 50: Sabbath Rest

God has shown Himself to be faithful to me and my family. It's given me time to write and do something of lasting value. I am grateful that through this work, I have the privilege of proclaiming the magnificence of my Lord and Savior, Jesus Christ. It has given me the chance to be true to the calling God gave me to write about my experiences with breast cancer. Through me, I hope other women can start to see His fingerprints in every aspect of their cancer journey. This has been part of His Sabbath rest for me.

The end of this book begins a new chapter for Dave and I, one where we step into our cancer-free, bent but not broken life together. We live to the fullest as we walk with the Lord. We have chosen to make this a new start, and it's our prayer for all of you who have come to the end of this book as well. We pray you too, will walk this path with Jesus and give Him the glory no matter what may come. Take your Sabbath rest in Him! Shalom!

✸ Devotional

There's an older song that I came across several years ago by a group called Selah. In the Bible, selah means to pause or reflect.

The title of the song is Press On:

When the valley is deep
When the mountain is steep
When the body is weary
When we stumble and fall

When the choices are hard
When we're battered and scarred
When we've spent our resources
When we've given our all

In Jesus' name, we press on
In Jesus' name, we press on
Dear Lord, with the prize

Day 50: Sabbath Rest

Clear before our eyes
We find the strength to press on

Brothers and sisters, I do not consider myself yet to have taken hold of it. But one thing I do: Forgetting what is behind and straining toward what is ahead, I press on toward the goal to win the prize for which God has called me heavenward in Christ Jesus. – Philippians 3:13-15

God bless you, my Pink Sisters and fellow cancer survivors, as you take your Sabbath rest and then in Jesus' name — press in and press on!

Prayer

Our loving Heavenly Father, there is no one like You. You have brought me this far and have faithfully walked with me every step of the way. No matter where I am in my journey or where You take me from here, I trust You. I depend on You to stay close to my heart, provide wisdom in the journey, and give me both peace and rest for my soul. Guide and direct me as I praise Your name in all circumstances. I pray in the matchless name of Jesus Christ, Amen.

> *Did you enjoy reading SOMEWHERE BETWEEN?*
> *Be sure to write a review on Amazon!*

Conclusion

As I look back on the last few years, I'm reminded of the uncertainty of life and the faithfulness of God. Whether we're navigating through cancer or some other life event, we're always somewhere between the past and future.

To be honest, after I finished writing this book, I put it away for several months and just wanted to keep healing and let that be my happily ever after. Unfortunately, it wasn't. In the months to follow, I experienced more scar breaks and infections, as well as the looming threat of skin grafts. After all this time, I'm still a rebel with ridiculous faith, looking back on what the Lord has done and continuing to grab hold of the promise for total healing. I have refused to relinquish more ground to the enemy or concede the victories Jesus made possible. To date, my scar has broken open three more times and has spontaneously healed before I could even get stitched. My skin now appears to be pink and healing normally. Praise God for this miracle!

I am more grateful today that I've ever been. How could a life-threatening illness accomplish that? Cancer has given me a deeper understanding of God's character and my identity in Christ alone. What God says about me, what He has done for me and what He has promised is imminently more important than anything else. He alone is Truth, and a malignancy will never define who I am. I am a beloved daughter, cancer or not, and a forever devoted follower of Jesus Christ. This is what sustains me and makes me incredibly grateful to be alive.

I am grateful for a tribe who loves, supports and challenges me to fulfill my God-given purpose while also allowing me to call them up to higher places for the Kingdom. I have experienced God's care in these mutually uplifting relationships and through them, have come to realize that I am never alone.

Cancer has made me grateful for a Christian mate who daily paints a picture of what sacrificial love looks like. During my illness, Dave showed me what it meant to be a true leader, protector, defender, and man of God. He stepped up to the plate and took each curve ball like a major league player. He continues to be my steady anchor in the storm, praying us through and loving me like no other — despite all my broken

Conclusion

pieces. Having cancer has helped me to see God through the words and actions of my husband and brought us to a place we may never have experienced if I had not been sick.

My gratitude has been birthed in the "between" times are where the Spirit does His best work. He grows me in ways I never thought possible and helps me to lay down who I am and pick up who He is. Recognizing cancer as a chronic condition rather than something that is "one and done" helps me live one day at a time and cope with the uncertainty of whether it will someday return. Jesus continues to encourage me with the words, "I am with you always, even until the end of the age," especially in the in-between times.

Now that my cancer treatment is complete, my biggest take away is an understanding that God's purposes are far greater than any problem. He always has and always will use everything for my good and His glory-even when I don't like it! II Corinthians 4:7-12 is correct in stating that "we have this treasure in jars of clay to show that this all-surpassing power is from God and not from us." I'm still a cracked pot, (for sure) but hopefully the light of the Lord will continue to shine through my life as I walk with Him.

The ups and downs of life are distinct but not unique and there's nothing He doesn't understand. Every story has its twists and turns, but they all have a purpose. My dance with the Lord continues to challenge me with new songs and steps, but I'm okay with that. I know He'll teach me as we go, and they will be as beautiful as He is.

With each day I am more convinced of His truth for all of us:

Allowing the pieces of our broken human condition to come into alignment with God's glorious design, is where we find the truest picture of who we are in the light of our magnificent Savior. Even when it means being somewhere between.

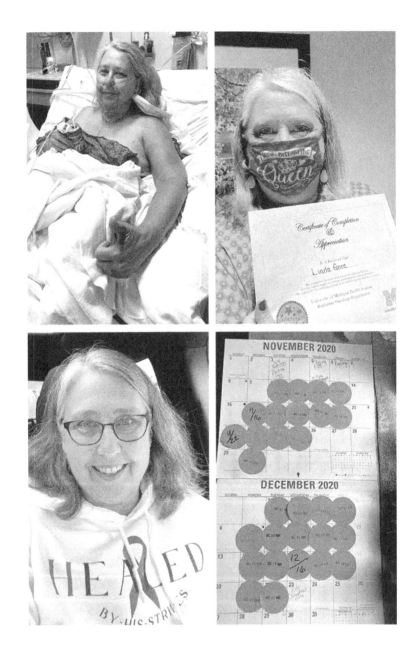

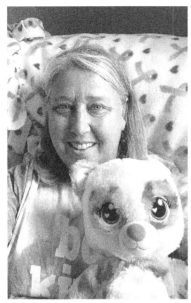
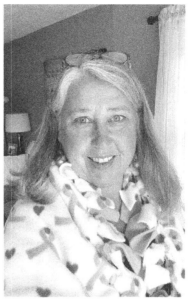
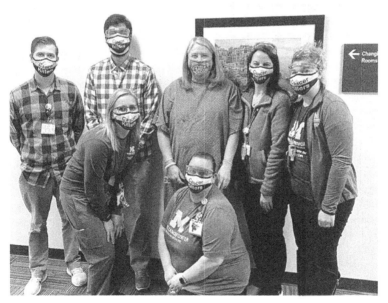

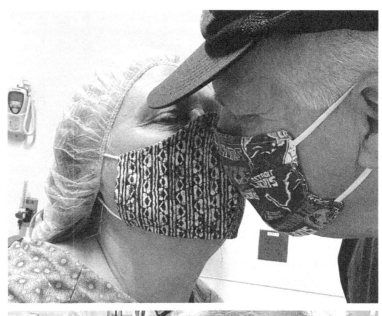
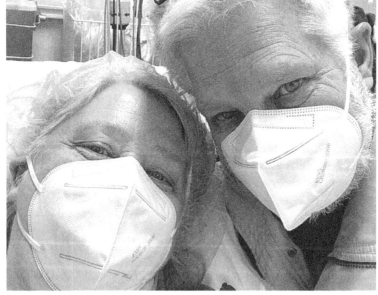

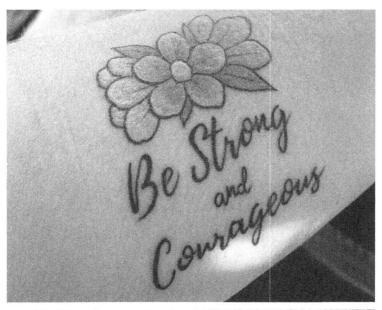
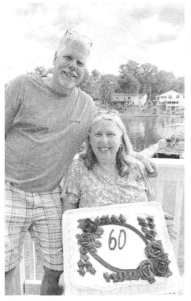
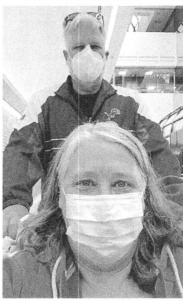

Appendix

How to Give Your Life to Jesus and Accept Him as Your Lord and Savior

When we are diagnosed with cancer, it brings mortality to the forefront of our lives. During times of crisis like this, we look for comfort, assurance and the hope that everything will be alright. The thing is, there's no real way to know whether we will physically survive cancer or succumb to it. That is the place where faith gets real. What you believe and who you believe in will be the difference between an eternity with God in Heaven or eternal separation from Him.

Knowing there is a God and knowing Jesus exists is not enough. You must have a personal relationship with God and accept Jesus Christ as your Lord and Savior if you want the assurance of being with Him forever.

You might be thinking, *That doesn't seem fair. Why do I have to accept Jesus to go to heaven? I'm a good person. I have certainly done my share of suffering with this cancer. Why wouldn't I go to Heaven if cancer gets me? A good God would welcome me into Heaven wouldn't He? I think after all this, I deserve to be there.*

While it's true that God loves us and wants an intimate relationship with us, the problem is that we're born sinful and our sin separates us from God. We're physically, mentally and spiritually broken. The Bible tells us there is nothing anyone can possibly do to fix that. In fact, we'd have to be perfect to have a relationship with a holy God —and obviously we're not! We might think we deserve Heaven after all the hell and suffering we've gone through with cancer, but the Bible teaches that we don't deserve anything from God. It's only because of His love and grace toward us that we have a chance to have an eternity with Him. John 3:16 says, *"For God so loved the world that He gave His only Son, that whosoever believes in Him should not perish, but have everlasting life."* Jesus paid the price to redeem or buy us back from our sin, and that's Good News!

Appendix

He did it with His perfect life's blood. Since we are sinful and can't redeem ourselves, the only way to restore that relationship is to accept the blood sacrifice of Jesus Christ, who became a substitute for the punishment we deserved. Jesus lived the perfect life we couldn't live, died the death we deserved so we could have the relationship with God that He wants to restore to us. If we refuse to accept Jesus, we refuse the only solution to our sin problem. If we accept Him, we get to be in heaven for eternity. That's a pretty good exchange and why the Gospel is called the Good News! Everyone dies physically, but spiritually we all have a choice about our eternal destination. Some choose Jesus and spend eternity together with God, while others reject Him and allow their sin to separate them from God for all eternity.

How can that be? Well, God, being perfectly loving, has devised a plan for us, from the beginning of time. Jesus wasn't an afterthought but part of the plan for our redemption all along. He wants to freely offer that gift of salvation and eternal life with Him to anyone who is interested. If you choose to accept His gift, it is freely given to you without condition. The

Bible says, *"If you confess with your mouth Jesus is Lord and believe in your heart that God raised Him from the dead, you will be saved"* (Romans 10:9). By believing and confessing, you are in essence accepting the free gift God has offered you. There's really no reason to wait. When cancer is involved, it becomes even more crucial to make a decision about your eternity. Why not accept Jesus? Why not give your life to Him? What is holding you back? What are you afraid of?" God loves you unconditionally and is waiting for you to come to Him. A story of faith like mine can be your story, too! If you are ready to dedicate your life to Christ and live as a child of God, if you are willing to trust Him with your today and tomorrow, all you have to do is go to Him in prayer and ask Him to take control. Prayer is just talking to God. You can talk to Him like you talk to anyone else. There is no special prayer or special ritual to go through. In order to make you more comfortable, you could read this prayer out loud as you commit your life to Jesus.

Appendix

Prayer of Salvation:

God, I know I have sinned and made mistakes. I confess I am guilty of missing the mark. I know Jesus, God's one and only Son, lived a perfect life on earth and died for me. I believe that His blood, shed on the cross, has paid the price for my sins, and I accept His sacrifice today. He has redeemed me; He forgives me and remembers my sin no more. I am grateful that from today I start my new life as a child of God. I acknowledge that I am unconditionally loved and accepted by my Lord and Savior. I invite You, Holy Spirit, to take control of my life and dwell within me, helping and guiding me in this new life I now live. Thank You, Jesus, for saving me and redeeming me. Thank You, Holy Spirit, for empowering me to live a holy life. Thank You, Father God, for loving me. Help me to love You and love others for the rest of my life. Lead me and guide me all the days of my life.

In Jesus' name, Amen.

If you prayed that prayer, you have crossed over from spiritual death to life no matter what your physical condition. You are now right with God. You have been bought with a price and you are redeemed. You are born again!

Today is your spiritual birthday!

Find a pastor, relative, and/or friend to share the Good News with! Or email me with the Good News and I will celebrate together with you.

Praise God and Welcome to the Family!

Lindy

Lindygoreministries@gmail.com

About The Author

Lindy Gore grew up in Cedar Rapids, Iowa, and was one of five siblings. Lindy taught students with special needs for more than twenty years while raising her two children, Ryan and Lacey. After a radical conversion to Christ in 1998, Lindy heard God calling her to mission and returned to graduate school to prepare for missionary life. Two years later, she completed a Master of Intercultural Studies degree at Fuller Theological Seminary and retired from teaching to pursue mission in Asia. Lindy lived, taught, and ministered throughout China for seven years. She also traveled internationally, ministering in Africa and Asia.

In 2015, Lindy returned to the United States, where she met and later married the love of her life, David Gore. After being diagnosed with invasive breast cancer in 2020, Lindy stepped back from her campus ministry with International students.

Lindy and Dave are active members of Radiant Church and serve together on the prayer team. Lindy has led a variety of small groups and uses her testimony to speak into the lives of others with cancer. When Lindy isn't hanging out with her adult children and six grandchildren, she and Dave can be found working together in their real estate business or DIYing a home project. They enjoy living on Goguac Lake in Battle Creek, Michigan, spending time with Dave's adult son, Austin, and their family and friends.

Notes